Dedication

This booklet is dedicated to the volunteer members of mountain rescue units all over the world. These modern day "Good Samaritans" give of themselves unselfishly so that their ill or injured fellow men may survive.

It is also dedicated to my mother, whose claim that I neglect her in order to spend time in the mountains may have validity.

Preface to the Thirteenth Edition

This is the fifteenth reprinting of this book since the initial 1,000 copies were published in 1965. Sales of the first 12 editions (two of the 12 editions underwent first and second printings) have totaled approximately 136,500 copies to date. My primary goal in writing this book has been, and is, dissemination of medical knowledge applicable to illness and injuries incurred in the wilderness. All backcountry users need information of this type before venturing into out-of-the-way places. Each new edition since the original publication 27 years ago has been updated by the addition of new "state of the art" medical information, and prior knowledge has often been rephrased to improve clarity.

Before each new edition, appropriate medical literature is reviewed, and knowledgeable physicians are asked to submit suggestions for improving the book. Constructive input from readers is also carefully considered.

Since space in this calculatedly small book is at a premium, usually only one method is presented for a given diagnostic or treatment procedure. The author believes the methods described are the safest and most appropriate for use by the average lay person when in wilderness conditions. A trained professional may elect to use other methods with equally good results. In several still-controversial areas of diagnosis or treatment, the method recommended is the one in concordance with current majority medical opinion. In all cases, the benefit/harm ratio of the recommendations has been very carefully considered. Still, sometimes there are no good answers, and one must make the best choice one can in a desperate situation!

This booklet was written primarily with the mountaineer in mind, but the material is equally useful for outdoorsmen and wilderness travelers of all interests, including hikers, backpackers, wilderness rangers, rock "hounds", hunters, high lake fishermen, cross-country skiers, canyoneers, trail riders,

MOUNTAINEERING MEDICINE

A Wilderness Medical Guide

13th edition

Fred T. Darvill, Jr., M.D.

Orthopedic Consultant- John A. Feagin, M.D.

Happy Hiking !
Fred Darvill, M.D.

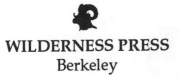

WILDERNESS PRESS
Berkeley

Acknowledgments

Over the years, constructive suggestions with regard to this booklet have been solicited from a number of physicians experienced in wilderness medicine. The author has not always accepted their advice, but all input from professional colleagues has been carefully considered. Doctors contributing to previous or current editions have included John Arnold, Otto Trott, William Halliday, Gene Mason, Earl Cammock, James Wilkerson, Herbert Hultgren, Charles Houston, Cameron Bangs, Gary Clancey, John Halsey, Rodman Wilson, Peter Hackett, Findlay Russell, Hugh Toomey, Robert Leach, and Earl Armbrust.

Illustrations by Marjorie Domenowske, Seattle, WA.

Thirteenth Edition 1992
Copyright © 1992 by Dr. Fred Darvill
Library of Congress Card Catalog Number 92-24834
ISBN 0-89997-155-5
Printed in the United States of America
Published by   Wilderness Press
                2440 Bancroft Way
                Berkeley, CA 94704
                (510)843-8080
                Write for free catalog

Library of Congress Cataloging-in-Publication Data

Darvill, Fred T., 1927-
    Mountaineering medicine : a wilderness medical guide / Fred T.
Darvill, Jr. ; orthopedic consultant, John A. Feagin. — 13th ed.
        p. cm.
    Includes bibliographical references and index.
    ISBN 0-89997-155-5
    1. Mountaineering—Accidents and injuries—Handbooks, manuals,
etc. I. Title.
RC1220.M6D37 1992
616.9'8—dc20   92-24834
                                                CIP

etc. It is primarily designed to be carried in the pack with the first-aid kit, but it is equally appropriate in the glove compartment of a backcountry car.

Part of the royalty income from the sale of this book is used to support mountain rescue units and part is donated to organizations promoting environmental preservation. In addition, royalties support organizations working toward the control of overpopulation and the prevention of nuclear war.

The first edition of *Mountaineering Medicine* was published by *Summit* magazine. The next eight editions reached print under the supervision of the Skagit Mountain Rescue Unit of Mt. Vernon, WA. In 1982, the author felt that the skills of a professional publisher would facilitate dissemination of the information contained herein, and an association was established with Wilderness Press. That organization has published the last four editions.

This book is written for the average lay reader. It is not a guide for health-care professionals. Paramedics, nurses, physicians and others desiring more advanced information should consult one or more of the professional publications listed in the Wilderness Medicine References at the back of this book.

For over three decades, my elderly mother has reluctantly shared me with the mountains. Hopefully she has come to understand that if I am sane, it is because I go to the mountains frequently. What I find in the high meadows, others find in church. All of us need to know where we feel closest to God!

John A. Feagin, M.D., a certified specialist in orthopedic surgery and Fellow of the American College of Surgeons, served as consultant for the accident and injury sections of this edition. Dr. Feagin has had extensive experience managing mountaineering and skiing injuries in the Tetons. His substantial contributions are acknowledged and appreciated.

Fred T. Darvill, Jr., M.D., F.A.C.P.
October 1992

Important!

Much of the information contained herein is part of the practice of medicine rather than standard first aid (e.g., use of potent medications such as morphine and antibiotics, reducing a dislocated shoulder). Using this information as recommended is more likely to benefit than to harm when injury or illness occurs in the wilderness far from a physician or hospital; however, these techniques should not be used by relatively untrained persons if professional assistance is close at hand. In other words, see a doctor if he is nearby, rather than attempting treatment based on the advice given in this publication.

Medicine, unlike physics, is an inexact science. Occasionally the best and most timely treatment does not produce the desired outcome. There are no guarantees in the practice of medicine, whether it is being practiced in a major hospital or in the remote mountains. This is particularly true when diagnoses must be made and treatment rendered far from a well-staffed and equipped modern facility. However, it is equally obvious that timely quality care, even under field conditions, is more likely to produce a favorable outcome than unsuitable and/or delayed therapy. Although the author has made every effort to provide reliable and appropriate approaches to the diagnosis and therapy of wilderness medical problems, the reader should realize there are no risk-free actions, either in a major hospital or in the wilderness.

Always carry these essentials while climbing or traveling in the wilderness; (1) map of the area; (2) compass; (3) flashlight; (4) waterproof matches, and a firestarter such as a candle or fire ribbon; (5) sun glasses; (6) sunscreen; (7) knife; (8) extra food; (9) extra clothing; (10) first-aid kit.

Introduction

Obviously, there is a vast difference between being ill or injured in the mountains many miles from the nearest physician's office or the nearest hospital, and having a similar illness or accident in a large city. It is therefore mandatory for every climber and backcountry traveler to know how to render proper medical treatment for ill and injured people until professional care can be obtained. Certainly on expeditionary climbing and ideally on every climb, a mountaineering physician should be included in the party. Even a fine physician, however, is limited in the care he can give by both the terrain and the available equipment.

Each climber should take a standard first-aid course and in addition acquire as much additional data on mountaineering medicine as possible; climbing physicians present data of this type in the climbing courses sponsored by various mountaineering clubs.

In addition, each climber should prepare for possible injury by being immunized routinely against tetanus (requires two to three injections initially, and then one injection every 10 years indefinitely), and desirably against typhoid, polio and diphtheria. (It is also possible presently to be immunized against Hepatitis B; the three required injections are expensive.) This immunization program can be accomplished when the mountaineer consults his family physician to obtain prescriptions for the medications in the first-aid kit which require a physician's authorization.

Excitement and tension after an accident may cause even a trained professional to function temporarily below his optimum level. Experience and knowledge are specific antidotes for nervousness at the scene of an accident. It is important to consider the most serious medical problems first, and to treat these conditions before proceeding to the management of less severe injuries or illnesses.

Implicit in the concept of "First Aid" is an anticipated delay time of 10-30 minutes from the time of injury, or from the development of major symptoms, until hospital admission. A similar accident or illness occurring on a major mountain or deep in the backcountry will on average require 48 hours before hospitalization can be achieved (longer in the Third World). Appropriate management of the wilderness emergency requires medical and logistic considerations not covered by standard Red Cross first-aid principles. Logical improvisation is the rule rather than the exception for providing the best possible medical management deep in the wilderness or high on a mountain.

Many nonmedical factors need to be carefully considered before determining the preferred management of illness or injury occurring far from a hospital. These include:

1. Weather—both current and predicted for the next 48 hours if known.
2. Ambient temperatures—current and anticipated; consider season of the year and wind-chill factor.
3. Time of day—remaining hours of daylight; is safe travel possible at night?
4. Party strength—number of persons on hand and their current physical capacities.
5. Medical skills of party members.
6. Communication abilities—travel time (distance and difficulty) to the nearest telephone or two-way radio.
7. Distance to the nearest evacuation location—road, helipad, etc.

8. Available materials carried by party members—tents, sleeping bags, first-aid kits, medications, stove, food, etc.
9. Availability of potentially useful materials on site—water, shelter, firewood, splint materials, etc.
10. On-site dangers—rockfall, avalanche, lightning, grizzly bears, etc.
11. Mental status—consider both the injured or ill person and the other party members.

These logistic considerations, when coupled with the data obtained by a quality history and physical examination, should lead to the formulation of an appropriate management plan that will maximize the likelihood of a favorable outcome.

Initial Accident Assessment

1. Above all else, keep calm and **THINK!** There is no emergency so urgent that ten to thirty seconds cannot be spent in thought. **THINK FIRST—THEN ACT!**
2. Carefully examine the patient in the position in which he is found (unless impractical due to other hazards, such as rockfall, avalanche and lightning). Do not move him until the severity of the injury has been determined.
3. Immediately and simultaneously evaluate heart action and breathing, and check for major blood loss. Note chest action. Check for heart beat (determine pulse in the arm or neck arteries). These three problems are the only cardinal medical emergencies that require immediate treatment!
4. Then examine for shock, head injury, fractures, dislocations, lacerations, and other injuries.

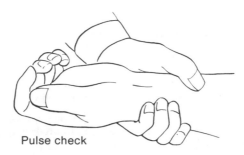

Pulse check

5. Comfort and reassure the injured person.
6. The head of the treatment team should be the individual with the greatest training in wilderness medicine. Immediately after the initial examination, he should give directions to other members of the climbing party to prepare medical supplies in order to institute prompt treatment. (In a small group, of necessity, all members of the climbing party become members of the treatment team. In a large group, the 3-5 medically most skilled climbers should care for the injured person.) He should also confer as soon as possible with the climb leader, since in addition to immediate treatment, decisions must be made regarding evacuation and/or summoning outside assistance. On both of these points, if in doubt it is better to be conservative and assume that the patient cannot be evacuated under his own power, and that additional assistance will be needed for definitive therapy and/or evacuation.
7. If the patient cannot be immediately removed from the area of the accident, an emergency camp should be established. The patient should be transported to a warm, dry camp site if possible, or if impossible,

firewood should be brought to the bivouac area. A fire
(or two fires between which the victim can be placed)
will keep the injured person warm, build morale, and
serve as a location marker for a rescue party.

Hemorrhage (Bleeding)

Significant bleeding must be controlled as soon as possible.
Stopping blood loss takes precedence over treatment of any
other problems, except cessation of breathing or heart beat,
which must be managed simultaneously.

*Almost all hemorrhage can be controlled by pressure
directly over the wound.* Immediately apply sterile 3 x 3
inch gauze dressings from the first-aid kit over the wound;
cover these with the cleanest available bulky cloth, and
apply constant firm pressure for 10 to 15 minutes. The
appropriate amount of pressure is the least amount
required to stop the bleeding.

Too little pressure will not halt blood loss; too much
pressure causes discomfort and may do further damage.
If initially bleeding is brisk, use the first available clean
fabric until sterile supplies are available. The risk of
infection is negligible compared to the risk of continued
blood loss.

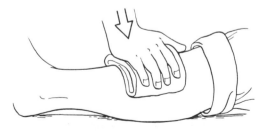

Direct pressure over bleeding wound

After the bleeding has stopped, remove the bulky cloth, leaving the sterile gauze in place (in order not to pull away the clot). Apply more sterile gauze if appropriate to cover the remainder of the wound; then wrap the area snugly, but not tightly, with an elastic bandage.

If significant blood loss has occurred, a patient who is without symptoms lying down may feel lightheaded when he stands up. After more extensive blood loss, consciousness may be lost if the person attempts to stand, and other signs of shock may develop. A patient with any of the above findings after appreciable blood loss should be evacuated supine (see section on shock for additional data).

Brisk bleeding from the scalp or extremities which has not been controlled after 10 minutes of firm direct pressure over the wound may require additional measures. "Pressure points" are locations where major arteries (blood vessels carrying blood from the heart to the body) may be effectively compressed against underlying bones and muscles. Occluding blood flow at these locations for 5-10 minutes may assist in controlling severe bleeding, in conjunction with continued use of local pressure applied to the wound.

Elevation of an extremity, in conjunction with the other more important methods of controlling bleeding noted above, may be helpful and is worth trying, unless other injuries to the limb make this supplemental technique inadvisable.

Bleeding associated with a fracture can often be controlled by splinting the arm or leg; an air splint is particularly useful for controlling blood loss from a severely fractured and lacerated extremity.

If significant bleeding from an extremity continues in spite of the use of the above techniques (this is more likely

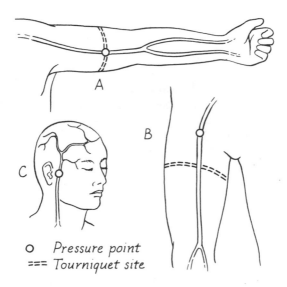

○ Pressure point
=== Tourniquet site

if blood was spurting from the wound with each heart beat before the pressure dressing was applied), the use of a tourniquet should be considered. Some authorities feel that tourniquets are more dangerous than helpful under any circumstances. However, the American Academy of Orthopedic Surgeons states as follows: "A properly applied tourniquet may be life-saving for a person whose bleeding from a major vessel is uncontrollable in any other way. Specifically, the tourniquet is useful in the patient who has sustained a traumatic amputation, either partial or complete, or in the patient for whom local pressure has failed."

The decision on whether to apply and, if used, when to release a tourniquet should be made by the most experienced person present after carefully considering all of the factors in the situation. Frequently, the decision to use a tourniquet involves a calculated sacrifice of the extremity in order to save the life of the individual.

Tourniquets are particularly hazardous when it is cold because of the likelihood of frostbite to the extremity deprived of warm blood. On the other hand, low environmental temperatures make shock more likely, and further blood loss predisposes to shock.

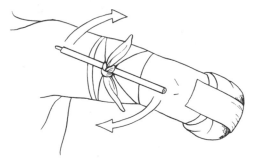

Application of tourniquet

Tourniquets may be improvised from any cloth or bandage material available; whatever is used should be several inches wide. Never use wire or other material that would cut through the skin. The tourniquet is applied to the upper part of the extremity between the torso and the wound. Note the time of application. The device is tightened by inserting any available long, firm object (metal rod, stick of wood, ice ax, etc.), and twisting this handle until sufficient pressure is produced to stop the bleeding. The ends of the "handle" must be well secured before the patient is transported. Unless the patient is in shock, the constricting device may be cautiously loosened one-half hour after application; the extremity should be elevated for several minutes before the tourniquet is released. If bleeding has stopped, the tourniquet should be removed. If bleeding resumes, the tourniquet should be immediately re-tightened sufficiently to stop bleeding. Further attempts at removal are probably inadvisable thereafter.

If shock due to blood loss exists, or is considered probable, any further bleeding may be so hazardous that the tourniquet should not be released under any circumstances until the patient reaches a hospital.

A tourniquet after application should never be covered with a bandage, since it may be overlooked if obscured. To alert others that the patient has a tourniquet, write "TK" on the patient's forehead, and on any identification tag attached to the patient; be sure the time of placement is noted also.

Traumatic amputations are a special situation. Since damage by the tourniquet to the extremity is no longer a consideration, the tourniquet is left in place continuously until the patient reaches the hospital (Life-endangering bleeding may not occur even with accidental amputation of an arm of leg, since the cut blood vessels retract into the muscle mass of the stump; if that occurs, the problem may respond to a firm compression dressing. However, if bleeding continues in spite of these measures, the tourniquet should be applied as close as possible to the amputation site.)

In desperate cases when all other techniques fail, it may be possible to grasp the spurting artery with the fingers and squeeze it closed to stop the bleeding; unfortunately, actively bleeding vessels are very slippery. More effective is seizing the blood vessel with a medical instrument called a hemostat and clamping it shut. This is a very effective method, but is often technically difficult, even for those with professional experience.

(See section on wounds re AIDS precautions.)

Wounds

Betadine (povidone-iodine 10% solution) is the preferred irrigating material for cleansing wounds of any size, but portability limits usage in the backcountry, since the amount that can be easily carried is inadequate for cleansing major wounds or open fractures. Betadine solution is available in 15 ml, 120 ml, and larger plastic bottles; these are bulky, and almost assuredly will spill eventually in the average pack. Foil packets of ointment and solution are available, but logistically also have limited value. Small Swab-Aid packets are easily portable, and well worth carrying for the cleansing of minor wounds. Single swab sticks in a plastic packet are also portable and relatively puncture proof. If Betadine is available, use it in place of the water and soap described in the next paragraph.

Wounds without appreciable bleeding should be gently washed with water that has been boiled and then allowed to cool to body temperature. Alternatively, drinking water treated with a Potable-Aqua tablet may be used if preboiled water is not available. Adding a bland soap to the water facilitates the removal of dirt and germs. After the soap has been washed out and the excess water removed (Betadine may be left in the wound), a dressing, desirably sterile, and certainly clean, is applied.

Gaping clean wounds may be closed with "butterfly dressings" when medical care is over 24 hours away. The tape is applied to one side of the wound, the wound pulled together, and the tape then stuck to the other side of the wound. Needless to say, the part of the "butterfly" in contact with the wound should be sterile. Butterfly dressings can be purchased commercially or can be made from adhesive tape. The central part of the device should not be sticky.

A grossly contaminated wound containing dirt, etc., should never be closed in the field. After gently removing as much dirt as possible, cover such a wound with a sterile dressing; delayed closure can take place in the hospital.

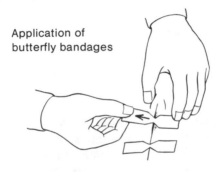

Application of
butterfly bandages

If doubt exists as to whether a wound is clean or not, consider it dirty and leave it open.

Minor or moderate clean wounds do not require antibiotic treatment. Grossly contaminated moderate wounds and major wounds (such as an open fracture) should receive antibiotic capsules if medical facilities are over six hours away.

Merthiolate, other forms of iodine and similar tissue poisons should never be placed in any wound.

"Sucking" chest wounds, where air is clearly moving into the chest with inspiration, should be covered immediately with an occlusive material applied sufficiently tightly to prevent air transfer.

Precautions to prevent the transmission of AIDS should be taken by rescuers when treating all bleeding wounds. Barriers to prevent skin, eye, or oral contact with blood should be utilized. The most important measure is to wear rubber gloves throughout, remove them cautiously to avoid blood contact, and wash hands promptly and thoroughly after removal. Masks, protective eye wear, and gowns or aprons are also advisable if they can be improvised.

Cessation of Respiration

Stoppage of breathing is a medical emergency requiring immediate treatment. In the mountains, accidents causing stoppage of respiration are uncommon. The usual causes are drowning or electrocution by lightning; severe crushing chest injuries may cause inadequate respiration, but seldom complete stoppage.·

The first step in treatment is to be sure that the "airway," the passage from mouth and nose to lungs, is clear. Remove mucus, water, dentures, etc. and be sure that the tongue has not be "swallowed." Use fingers and/or gravity to extricate materials blocking the passage of air. The neck must be extended (head pulled back), and the jaw pulled forward (see diagram) to maximize the patency of the airway.

Mouth-to-mouth artificial ventilation is without question the method of choice for dealing with respiratory arrest (cessation of breathing). The two drawbacks of mouth-to-mouth resuscitation are that it is aesthetically unpleasant and there is a small risk of transmitting any mouth or general infections that the victim may have (such as herpes or AIDS). Nonetheless, with a life at stake, most rescuers are willing to accept the oral contact in spite of the above liabilities. (The back [prone]-pressure arm lift [Holger-Nielsen] method of artificial respiration, as taught in first-aid and life-saving classes 35-40 years ago, is archaic, and is no longer recommended. However, rescuers unwilling to accept mouth-to-mouth contact should familiarize themselves with and utilize this method, or alternatively carry a device, such as the Laerdal Pocket Mask, which permits mask-to-mouth ventilation without risk of infection.)

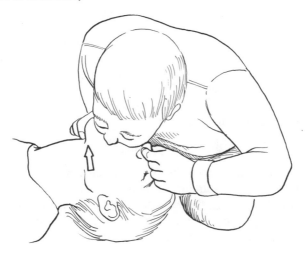

Mouth-to-mouth resuscitation technique

Technical instructions follow: If available, an oral-pharyngeal airway is inserted. The operator takes a deep breath and simultaneously closes the patient's nostrils with one hand; he then makes firm contact with his mouth over the patient's mouth so that no air escapes, and exhales deeply. The chest of the patient should obviously expand during this procedure; the patient's jaw may need to be pulled forward to open the airway. Good skin color and adequate chest motion indicate the procedure is effective; a blue color to the skin and failure of the chest to move indicate an immediate need to recheck the airway and the technique. Continue until effective spontaneous respiration resumes, or until death is obvious.

If you are unable to ventilate an unconscious person, or if you have witnessed a choking episode, assume airway obstruction with a foreign body. The Heimlich maneuver of subdiaphragmatic abdominal thrusts should be performed standing in a conscious patient, or supine if the victim is unconscious. Lifting the tongue and jaw and sweeping the back of the throat to remove any foreign body present are actions used in conjunction with the Heimlich maneuver in an unconscious victim. These techniques are taught in the standard CPR course, advisable for everyone.

Cessation of Heart Action

In cases of lightning strike (electric shock) or heart attack, both respiratory action and heart action may suddenly cease. In these cases, mouth-to-mouth respiration and restoration of heart action must be accomplished immediately (irreversible brain damage occurs in 4-8 minutes).

Place the patient on his back over a firm support. Kneel beside the patient and place the heel of one hand over the lower breast bone; place the other hand crosswise on top of the first (lower) hand. Depress the breast bone about 1.5-2 inches toward the spine 80 times a minute. Use body weight to provide pressure. Release weight completely between strokes. Continue until a physician is present or until futility is evident after one hour.

A second person simultaneously clears the airway and inserts an oral-pharyngeal airway if available. Mouth-to-mouth lung ventilation is then performed when the heart is not being massaged. With two rescuers, after every five heart compressions one lung expansion maneuver is performed. Heart compression is then resumed, and this cycle is repeated thereafter. If only one rescuer is present, after every 15 heart compressions the lungs are inflated twice.

Space does not permit a more detailed description of CPR techniques. Considerable practice is necessary to become and remain competent in these procedures; special courses in cardio-pulmonary resuscitation (CPR) are easily available. Instruction every two years is desirable to maintain appropriate skill levels.

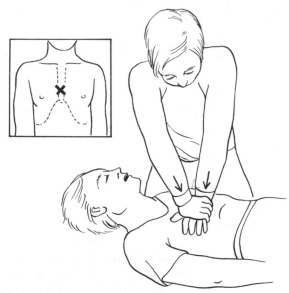

Position for external heart massage

Shock

After treatment of hemorrhage, respiratory difficulty and heart stoppage, the next priority is to assess for shock and treat it if present. Shock is a condition of acute circulatory collapse; it is most commonly caused by substantial blood loss, but can also occur following an injury without blood loss, due to a derangement of the blood-vessel control system. Symptoms of shock are pallor and clamminess of the skin, low blood pressure, rapid feeble pulse, shallow rapid breathing, sweating, restlessness, anxiety, nausea and vomiting, and sometimes partial or complete loss of consciousness. Shock may follow even minor injuries. It may be intensified by fear or by rough handling. The shock state can actually be more serious than the initial injury. It is appropriate to assume that shock exists following every accident until proven otherwise. Shock usually occurs within a few minutes following an accident, but it may develop as long as several hours later.

The following measures are used both to prevent and to control shock:

1. Place the patient flat on his back; if shock persists, raise the legs and thighs while maintaining the torso supine.
2. Keep the patient warm with all available clothing; replace wet clothing if possible. A patient in mild shock can still produce body heat, so that clothing will prevent heat loss. A patient in more severe shock loses the capacity to produce body heat; under these circumstances, no amount of clothing will maintain normal or restore subnormal body temperature. Hypothermia and irreversible shock then occur, and death ensues. Therefore, in cases of severe shock,

external heat must be applied, but the body must not be overheated or burned. The ideal heat source in the field is the body heat produced by other normal persons. One, two or more climbers should be enclosed in a "cocoon" of all available material (clothes, sleeping bags, etc.) with the patient in order to return body temperature to normal as rapidly as possible. Skin-to-skin contact is the most rapid way of transferring body heat.

If circumstances are such that body heat from other climbers is impractical, external heat from other sources should be added with appropriate precautions to prevent burns and gross overheating. The central body area (torso) should be warmed initially; application of heat to the extremities only may worsen the shock state (see the section on hypothermia). Obviously, in any shock state, further heat loss should be prevented.

3. Control accessory problems:

    a. Prevent further blood loss.

    b. Relieve pain with codeine or with an injection of morphine (the latter is preferred if available, provided that a significant head injury is not present).

    c. Handle the patient gently to prevent further injury, pain and apprehension.

    d. Splint fractures as soon as possible.

    e. Be sure the airway remains open at all times.

    f. Solid food should be avoided until the shock state has completely resolved; one climbing physician feels that warm, sweetened fluids by mouth are helpful during recovery if the injured person can swallow, is not nauseated, and does not have an abdominal injury.

Head and Spine Injuries

Head, neck and spine injuries are the most serious disasters which confront the alpine first-aider. The brain and spinal cord are both delicate and vital to life; rough handling or incorrect positioning may cause additional injury or death. Since a sequence of correct treatment is difficult to remember, carrying a booklet such as this or written notes to refresh the memory is often of great assistance when confronted with difficult decisions which must be made under wilderness conditions.

Head Injuries

Prevention is better than treatment; wear a hard hat!

Bruises, abrasions, scratches, and cuts of the scalp and forehead are managed as are wounds elsewhere. The magnitude of these superficial injuries does not well predict the likelihood of harm to the brain.

The crucial factor with regard to head injuries is whether or not the brain is damaged. The following guidelines are helpful.

1.   Negligible or no brain damage: The involved person is never unconscious, but may complain of being dazed or stunned or of "seeing stars;" ability to think rationally is never lost.

2.   Mild to moderate brain damage (concussion): A temporary loss of consciousness occurs, arbitrarily defined as lasting from a few seconds to 10 minutes. The severity of the injury is roughly proportional to the duration of unresponsiveness. There may be substantial mental malfunction (loss of memory and/or confusion) lasting from a few minutes to 5-6 hours after awakening occurs. Minimal abnormalities may persist for several

weeks. The longer substantial confusion persists, the greater the possibility of a significant brain injury. With most concussions, there is no permanent brain damage.

3.   Moderate to severe brain damage: Prolonged unconsciousness (coma) indicates more serious harm to the brain (laceration or bruising of brain tissue; bleeding within the skull). Evacuation by helicopter (less desirably by stretcher) is mandatory under these circumstances. Skull fracture frequently, but not invariably, is associated with major brain damage. The following findings suggest skull fracture or serious brain damage:

a.   Bleeding from ears, nose, and mouth if not due to local injury.

b.   Clear, watery fluid draining from ears or nose.

c.   Unequal pupils—one pupil larger than the other—particularly if the larger pupil does not get smaller when a bright light is flashed on it.

d.   Loss of muscle power or sensation in any area.

e.   Prolonged unconsciousness or semiconsciousness.

When confronted with a head injury, first control obvious bleeding from the scalp by local pressure as described under control of hemorrhage. If the patient is conscious, evaluate his judgment and factual knowledge (Where are you? What day is it? Who is President?). If judgment and factual knowledge are normal, the patient is alert, and none of the above signs is present, test coordination and balance by a trial walk with a climber on either side of the patient. If the trial walk shows no abnormalities, the patient may walk out under his own power, preferably without a heavy load. He should be assisted if necessary, and observed closely until professional attendance is available.

(Delayed   serious   bleeding   inside   the   skull

occasionally follows injuries initially considered mild. Clinically this is manifested by progressive decline in brain function after initial improvement. Because of this possibility, most outings should be aborted promptly after a concussion, even if a full recovery appears to have occurred initially; this is particularly true if the patient complains of headache following the injury.)

No specific treatment is available in the field for brain damage. Patients with evidence of major brain injury must be rapidly transported to the nearest hospital. Morphine should not be used if harm to the brain is suspected or definite. The time of injury and the progression of symptoms should be transmitted to the physician who will assume professional responsibility for the injured person.

Vomiting in an unconscious or stunned malfunctioning patient requires immediate action to prevent vomited material from entering the windpipe! Turn the patient onto his side or face down; lift the mid portion of the body (the pelvic bones provide handholds), so that the chest is higher than the mouth. Maintain the patient in this position until vomiting has ceased, and all of the regurgitated material has been cleared from the back of the mouth and throat.

Crucial to the management of the unconscious patient is the maintenance of the airway (the route through which the air passes from mouth and nose to lungs). Keep the jaw pulled forward (i.e., chin out). Use an oral-pharyngeal airway if available. If equipment to maintain the airway is lacking, a safety pin can be passed through the tip of the tongue, and affixed to the lower lip, or pulled farther forward and anchored to the chest with string and tape. This keeps the tongue from falling backward and blocking the airway.

Spine Injuries—neck (cervical)

Neck and head injuries often co-exist. Possible injuries of both areas should be evaluated concomitantly:

1. If the patient is conscious, determine if neck pain is present. An alert, nonparalyzed person with a significant injury will tend to keep the neck immobile, since movement increases pain.

2. If the patient is unconscious, it is best to assume that there is a significant neck injury as well as a head injury.

3. In an alert patient without other serious injuries, test for evidence of spinal-cord damage by asking the patient to move his arms or legs, and by determining whether there is any loss of sensation in the torso or extremities. Paralysis or "numbness" suggests that the spinal cord has already been damaged, and mandates extremely careful handling to prevent further irrevocable loss of nervous tissue.

4. If in doubt about the presence of a neck fracture, it is safest to assume one is present.

5. Treatment: It is essential that the patient be evacuated with an *absolute minimum* of neck motion. During any movement of the injured person by rescuers, the neck should be pulled gently away from the body, maintaining the neck in a normal position to the extent possible (neither bent forward nor arched backward). The patient's head, neck and body should be moved in unison, and movement should not be attempted until sufficient manpower is available to move the injured person in this manner. Once on the

stretcher (or a temporary alternative), the neck should be immobilized; a small pad beneath the neck is helpful to keep the head in the correct position. Additional support should be applied around the neck and head to prevent motion in any direction during transport.

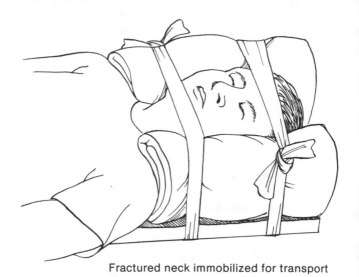

Fractured neck immobilized for transport

Spine Injuries—back (thoracic or lumbar)

Direct injury to the back is the most common cause of fractures; a broken backbone can also occur when a person lands on his feet or buttocks after a substantial fall. Severe persistent back pain following either of these types of accident strongly suggests a back fracture.

The patient should be evaluated in a similar manner as with neck fracture, by testing for both muscle use and loss of sensation. Again, if a back fracture cannot be excluded, assume it is present. *If in doubt always err on the safe side! Extremely careful evacuation is mandatory with suspected neck and back fractures; permanent damage to the spinal cord may occur as a result of inappropriate transport or treatment.*

Treatment: Again, the patient's body and neck must be moved in unison with the legs and back kept in a straight line and the back extended (arched backward).

A pad under the mid portion of the back will maintain the arch in the stretcher. The stretcher should be kept rigid and the arched position maintained until professional attendance is available.

A patient with a back injury can be moved quickly and fairly safely from a dangerous area, such as an active avalanche slope, by carrying him face down in a tightly stretched blanket, tent or tarp.

In summary, if back or neck fracture is suspected,

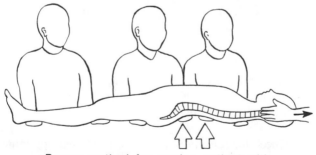

Proper method for moving patient with suspected neck or back fracture

immobilize the spine; also pad bony prominences, and remove material from pockets to prevent any pressure injury. Evacuate by helicopter if at all possible. (For health professionals: If paralysis is present or spinal-cord injury is thought probable, intravenous dexamethasone 10-15 mg. is desirable, particularly if it can be given within the first 4 hours after injury.) Less desirably, the drug can be given orally in a dose of 12-16 mg. (3-4 tablets of the 4 mg. strength).

Fractures

Fractures may be classed into two groups:

a.   Closed (simple)—where the bone is broken but the skin is not torn.
b.   Open (compound)—where a portion of the bone has protruded through the skin (note—the bone may protrude and then re-enter the body, leaving only a visible wound; a fresh wound and signs suggestive of fracture should be considered an open fracture).

The following findings suggest fracture:

1.   Deep pain at the point of injury.
2.   Tenderness localized over a bone at the site of injury.
3.   Obvious deformity of the affected area.
4.   Inability to use the affected area without extreme pain or inability to bear weight on it.
5.   A grating or rasping sensation noted with the rescuer's hand lightly held over the affected area when motion is attempted.

Check for sensation, motor function, and appearance initially, again following splinting, and periodically at regular intervals thereafter. There is disagreement among authorities whether it is wiser to keep a fractured extremity elevated at a level higher than the body (heart), or whether it should be left at approximately heart level. There is agreement that the injured part should not be dependent (below the level of the main portion of the body).

Field treatment of an arm or leg fracture is to splint the limb with the most practical available material. In general, one should splint both the joint above and the joint below the fracture. If the extremity is bent, gentle traction will often allow it to be straightened and splinted.

Open fractures require gentle but thorough washing to remove dirt and other foreign materials. (See cleansing instructions in Wound section.) When the wound is completely cleansed, a sterile dressing is applied. No attempt is made to close the wound. Unless hospitalization can be achieved within 1-2 hours, antibiotics should be administered in high doses (cephradine one gram every 6 hours).

Pain control with appropriate medication is important. Above timberline, splint materials are scarce and a good deal of ingenuity is required to immobilize a fracture. Ice axes or uninjured parts of the patient's own body may be the only splints available.

Plastic air splints, which are light and easily transportable, are excellent for immobilizing forearm, wrist, and ankle injuries, but less useful for fractures of the thigh and the upper arm. Another asset is that the pressure provided by the splint may assist in controlling bleeding from open wounds. These devices, however, do have

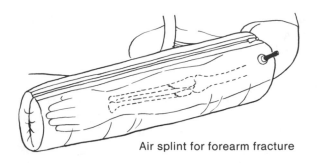

Air splint for forearm fracture

several drawbacks: 1) Punctures are not uncommon, with resultant loss of immobilization (the leaks, if located, can be patched with scotch tape). 2) Overinflation can substantially reduce blood flow into the limb; the splinted limb must be carefully watched, and pressure reduced if the skin turns blue or white, or pain worsens. In addition, if transportation is prolonged and/or the ambient temperature is cold, it is wise to release the air pressure intermittently when extremity movement is not likely. Also remember that with a significant change in altitude, the splint should be checked for over-inflation or deflation; 3) The plastic will stick to burned or abraded areas; open wounds should be dressed before the air splint is applied.

Structural aluminum malleable (SAM) splints have recently become available. These metal strips with a plastic coating can be rolled up like a bandage, or stored flat in a small space, and easily carried. When folded into a "structural bend" longitudinally, the strip becomes quite rigid. They are washable, and can be reused. X-rays can be taken through the material easily. In short, these splints are efficient, inexpensive, and portable.

The following points are important in the management of specific fractures: *Jaw fractures:* tape the jaw to the rest of the face or scalp (obviously inadvisable with concomitant nasal obstruction or tendency to

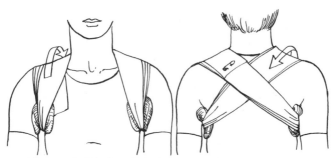

Figure-of-eight bandage for immobilizing a fractured collar bone

vomiting). If prolonged delay in reaching medical assistance is anticipated, leave a small opening to permit the ingestion of fluids. *Fractures of the collar bone:* Immobilize, using a figure-of-eight bandage around both shoulders. *Fractures of the upper arm:* Bind the arm to the chest by the use of an improvised sling and swath; cloth, elastic bandages or adhesive tape may be used.

Forearm and wrist fractures are best treated with the air splint if available; if not, apply a splint made from whatever material is available to the inner side of the arm, and support the arm in a sling thereafter.

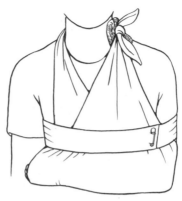

Sling and swath for immobilization of an upper
arm fracture or a dislocated shoulder

Fractures of the hand or fingers may be treated by
placing a small bit of clothing in the palm of the hand, and
having the victim make as much of a fist as pain will
permit; then wrap the hand in this position with an elastic
bandage. A fractured rib may be effectively treated by the
use of sufficient codeine or morphine to obtain relief of
pain. If multiple fractures exist or pain is very severe, the
ribs may be taped with several overlapping strips of 3-inch
tape which start beyond the midline on the uninvolved side
in front and extend beyond the midline on the uninvolved
side in back. One to three elastic bandages snugly applied
around the chest may also give relief of pain. Fractures of
the pelvis are usually quite painful; when there is
concurrent injury to the bladder or to the tube between the
bladder and the outside, there may be inability to urinate,
or passage of blood in the urine. In these situations, fluid

intake should be restricted. Pelvic fractures and leg fractures can be treated by tying the legs together. Place appropriate padding material between the extremities; then apply immobilizing material above and below the knees and above the ankles. A long splint from the waist to the ankle may increase immobility. Fractures of the upper leg are best treated with a Stokes litter and with one of the various traction splints (Hare; Thomas; Sager; Kendrick).

If these devices are unavailable, use the technique described above, or alternatively use any available rigid material to construct a "jerrybuilt" splint (see the diagram, where an ice ax is used for support). Fractures of the lower leg and ankles are best treated with the air splint or with splints from any appropriate material.

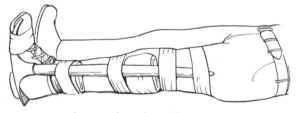

Ice-axe long leg splint

Circulatory impairment should be avoided during the splinting process. Particular care must be used when fractures (or severe sprains) are suffered under excessively cold conditions. A minor obstruction of circulation under these circumstances will predispose to frostbite. A splinted extremity must be observed carefully until a hospital is reached. If there is evidence of blocked circulation (pain at other than the site of injury; numbness and tingling; blueness or whiteness of tissues), the splint and bindings must be immediately adjusted.

Dislocations, Sprains and Strains

Dislocations

A dislocation is the displacement of the head of a bone from its socket. The shoulder is the most commonly dislocated joint. A dislocated shoulder is painful at rest, and discomfort accentuates substantially if the arm is moved; the shoulder appears pointed rather than rounded. Often the head of the arm bone can be felt in the arm pit. The preferred method of treatment, if medical aid is relatively accessible, is to bind the arm to the chest wall using an elastic bandage or adhesive tape (see sling-swath diagram) and seek medical assistance. If medical aid is a great distance away or the terrain precarious, reduction (replacing the head of the upper arm bone in its socket) of the dislocated shoulder can be attempted. Ideally, only trained personnel should attempt this procedure, since permanent damage can be caused by improper treatment.

If there is any reason to suspect a simultaneous fracture of any of the shoulder bones, socket reduction should not be attempted. On the other hand, a person whose dislocated shoulder has been put back in place may well be able to walk out rather than having to be evacuated.

Muscle relaxation facilitates reduction of a dislocation. This can be achieved through a combination of traction, massage of the muscles about the dislocated joint, and vocal assurance.

Medicine to relieve pain before attempting reduction may also be helpful. Two aspirin, 60 mgs. of codeine, and perhaps one 0.125 mg. Halcion tablet can be given by mouth one hour beforehand. If morphine is available, it can be given by a professional by vein a few minutes beforehand; given under the skin, it requires at least half an hour to be effective.

The patient should be instructed to relax the muscles around the shoulder as much as possible, regardless of which method of reduction is used.

Since involuntary muscle spasm worsens as time passes, the sooner the dislocation can be corrected, the better.

The simplest method involves finding a suitable rock, the cut end of a large log or a similar location. Have the patient lie prone on whatever is available so that his injured arm can hang over the side. Tie about 15 lbs. of weight to the arm at the elbow (20 lbs. for very large people; 10 lbs. for small people). Pad the attachment so

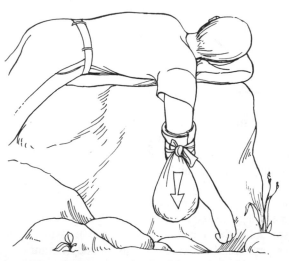

The safest way to reduce a dislocated shoulder

that undue pressure is not put on nerves or blood vessels. (If the weights will not stay on the elbow, the wrist can be used if there is enough space for the arm to descend that far.) Let the weighted arm hang down for about 15 minutes; during this time, the muscles should fatigue enough to allow the upper arm bone to slip back into normal position. This method is probably the safest way to deal with this condition.

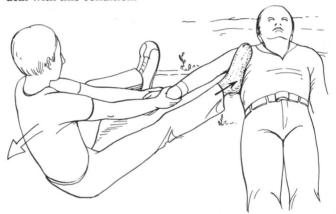

Another way to reduce a dislocated shoulder

If a suitable location cannot be found, or weights cannot be devised from available materials, find a fairly level area and place the patient on his back. The helper then sits alongside, and places a stockinged foot on the chest wall near (but never in) the arm pit; substantial steady traction is then applied along the patient's-arm-rescuer's-leg axis, counterforcing with the helper's leg. The person doing the reduction should keep his arms extended, and simply lean backward, thus using body weight to apply the necessary force. After 10-15 minutes, the head of the arm bone will often slip back into its socket spontaneously.

After the dislocation has been corrected, a sling and swath should be applied and left in place until professional help has been obtained.

Sprains

An injury to a joint causing stretching or tearing of supporting ligaments is called a sprain. Pain, swelling, and loss of function are usual symptoms. It is often difficult to differentiate a severe sprain from a fracture without the aid of x-rays.

The most common sprain in mountaineering is to the ankle joint. The primary consideration in emergency management is to prevent any further damage until definitive diagnosis and treatment can be obtained.

For a mild-to-moderate sprain, as indicated by slight pain and swelling, wrap the ankle with an elastic bandage* and tighten the boot to provide external support. The patient can usually walk out under his own power (with help over rough or difficult terrain); an ice ax, staff, or improvised crutch can be used to partially bear weight, thus sparing the involved limb.

For a severe sprain, diagnosed by the presence of major discomfort, substantial swelling, and a blue-purple

---

*(Place 2-3 turns around the ankle with the bandage under tension; then wrap a figure 8 between the ankle and the mid portion of the foot; the heel is excluded if properly applied. Secure with clips or a safety pin located in an area where body weight or boot pressure will not cause distress.)

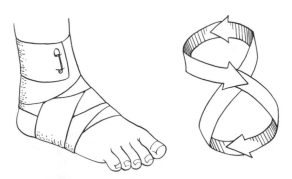

"Figure 8" application of elastic bandage
to treat ankle sprain

discoloration beneath the ankle bones 12-24 hours after the injury, transportation without weight bearing on the involved leg must be provided. Before and during evacuation, the extremity should be elevated to reduce swelling. The elastic bandage should be applied and the boot retained for support, but the boot should not be so tight that developing swelling would impair circulation, particularly if the ambient temperature is low (40°F or below). Aspirin and, if needed, codeine can be used to control pain.

If in doubt as to severity, err on the safe side and evacuate without weight bearing.

Apply cold (snow, cool water compresses, etc.) to the involved area for the first 24 hours in an effort to reduce swelling.

Strains

A strain is a rupture of the fibers of a muscle. The pain is usually localized over the mid portion of the extremity rather than in the region of a joint. Localized tenderness is present. Appropriate treatment is the application of cold for the first 24 hours, the control of pain, and the avoidance of painful activity.

The Acutely Painful Joint (overuse injury)

Repetitive vigorous activities, such as hiking and climbing, can cause various "overuse" problems, including inflammation of tendons (tendinitis), of lubricating sacs (bursitis), and of joints (arthritis). These conditions cause pain, swelling and sometimes redness in the area of the involved joint or tendon; the discomfort is often severe enough to be disabling if the knee or ankle is involved. Common examples include tendinitis or bursitis of the shoulder, Achilles tendinitis of the ankle, patellar tendinitis of the knee, and chondromalacia patella (irritation of the underside of the knee cap).

These conditions are best treated with approaches that diminish inflammation. Rest the involved area if possible. The application of cold materials may be helpful. Clothing dipped in cold water, or packed with snow, may be applied to the painful area intermittently; a reasonable schedule is for 15-20 minutes every 3-4 hours. Moderate discomfort will usually respond to aspirin (or, less desirably, Tylenol) in doses of two tablets every four hours. Pain not controlled by aspirin may respond to ibuprofen; this drug is now available without a prescription in 0.2 gram strength (trade names include Advil and Nuprin). The average-sized person will need to take two tablets four times a day. Both drugs may cause stomach upset as a side effect; taking the pills with food lessens the likelihood of indigestion.

Long downhill walks are the most common causes of these problems; if a party member is known to be prone to develop these difficulties, it is best to break up sustained downhill marches if possible. Using an ice ax, staff, or stick can help avoid the downhill impact which causes increased symptoms with overuse injuries of the lower extremities.

Frostbite

Frostbite, or freezing of the tissues, most commonly affects the body areas exposed to the elements (face, hands or feet). Subjective symptoms in sequence usually include a feeling of coldness that gradually becomes painful; then, as freezing progresses, both the pain and cold feeling disappear, and are replaced by a loss of sensation, a feeling as if the part did not exist. Objectively, in the early stages there may be no obvious change whatsoever, or the body part may be cold, white, or purple-tinged, or may appear hard (like meat kept in a deep freeze). Blisters, redness and black scabs are late changes.

Frostbite is usually preventable! Handling cold metal with unprotected hands should always be avoided. The proper protection of the feet with appropriate socks and boots is mandatory. The boots must be well fitted; tight laces or crampon straps must not be allowed to impair the inflow of warm blood to the feet. Cramped positions that block circulation should be avoided (e.g., move around in the snow cave). Wet socks increase heat loss greatly; socks should be kept dry if possible, or else changed whenever damp.

Gloves are indispensable for protecting exposed hands. A parka hood and face mask (balaclava) restrict heat loss from the head and face. Of even greater importance is the conservation of heat in the core of the body; if the temperature of the torso falls, the body automatically shunts blood away from the arms and legs in order to provide warmth to the more essential central organs. For this reason, as experienced mountaineers know, the addition of extra clothing to the torso will result in the warming of cold hands and feet.

Incipient frostbite (where the flesh is very cold, but no tissue damage has occurred), and first-degree frostbite (minor tissue damage is present) should be treated by warming the extremity against the warm skin of a companion (abdomen; armpit). More severe frostbite should not be treated until facilities for rapid rewarming are available. A climber may walk many miles on frozen feet, but once rewarming has been performed, he becomes a litter case. Rapid rewarming is achieved by immersing the cold-damaged body parts in water at 104-108 degrees F. (40-42 degrees C.); most authorities recommend the use of a thermometer, believing the temperature must be exact. However, in a crisis, one can test the water temperature by immersion of a normal hand. The water should be comfortably warm but should not burn the test hand. Severe pain occurs shortly after rewarming and therefore medication for pain relief should be available when rewarming is performed. Continue the soaking until flushing occurs in the tips of the fingers or toes, or for one hour, whichever is shorter. After the rewarming, the extremities should be handled gently to avoid further injury. Careful cleansing with a germicidal soap, use of padded sterile dressings, splinting, and observation for concomitant dehydration are indicated. Ideally, rewarming should be performed in a hospital where this equipment is available. If rewarming is done in the field, hospitalization must be effected as soon as possible.

Refreezing after rewarming causes great damage, and should be prevented at all costs.

Two other things should NOT be done:

1. The temperature of the frostbitten area should not be raised significantly above body temperature, such as warming by a fire.
2. The injured part must never be rubbed, especially not with snow, or treated roughly.

Both of these misguided efforts to help invariably increase the injury and cause further damage to already devitalized tissues.

Exposure (hypothermia)

This problem occurs when weather conditions are such that body heat is lost more rapidly than it can be produced. Body temperature falls first in the extremities, then in the central "core" areas; when irreversible changes due to low temperature in vital organs develop, death occurs.

As with most wilderness medical problems, prevention is more important than treatment. Individuals particularly susceptible to hypothermia are those of thin body build (usually male) who lack sufficient body fat immediately beneath the skin to insulate them adequately.

The two circumstances of greatest danger are the combination of physical exhaustion and wet clothing. Failure to eat is a contributory cause. This combination of conditions should be avoided at all costs, since mental deterioration can occur very rapidly under these circumstances, leaving the individual unable to make rational judgments. Death can occur in a surprisingly short time (a few hours) even in temperatures well above freezing, particularly if it is windy.

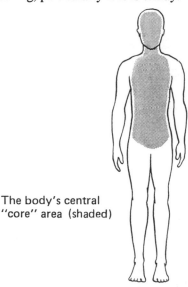

The body's central "core" area (shaded)

The following points of prevention are therefore emphasized. (1) Carry effective waterproof external garments and use them immediately when the weather deteriorates. (2) Bivouac before exhaustion occurs and construct the most effective practical shelter. (3) Carry extra food; eat frequently, particularly starches and sugars. (4) Keep as warm as possible with a fire or by huddling together to conserve body heat. (5) Wear appropriate clothing if adverse weather is probable (polypropylene or other synthetic underwear; pile or wool outer garments; waterproof parka and rain pants). Closed-cell foams, such as Ensolite, are very effective insulators; clothing containing these materials may become more available as time passes. (6) Drink warm liquids, both to prevent dehydration and to supply heat.

Hypothermia is common following head injuries, blood loss (especially if there is associated shock), and prolonged immobilization (as with a fracture) in a cold environment.

Symptoms (subjective sensations) and signs (observable abnormalities) develop sequentially in the average patient as body heat is progressively lost. The usual symptom complex may be significantly modified by special circumstances, particularly nutritional state, medication use, and activity level during exposure to cold.

Temperature 91°-98°F (33°-37°C): Early on, the victim will feel cold. The skin may show "goose bumps"; shivering begins, and becomes progressively more marked as body temperature falls. The body begins to feel cold to the touch; pulse and respiration become more rapid; paleness due to the constriction of superficial blood vessels is usually present. The victim may appear apathetic, lethargic and withdrawn. (When hiking or climbing, the hypothermic person may fall behind the rest of the group.) When body temperature falls to the low 90s, confusion and lethargy worsen, and inappropriate behavior may occur. Victims may urinate in their clothing. Mental activity becomes sluggish, speech is slowed, judgment is lost, and memory fails. Shivering stops (the cessation of shivering is a good sign when body temperature is rising but an ominous sign when body temperature is falling).

Temperature 86°-90°F (30°-32°C): Muscles become rigid, gross incoordination occurs; mental activity declines rapidly; the patient may become completely unresponsive (coma).

Temperature 80°-85°F (27°-29°C): Progressively deepening coma, muscle rigidity, progressive fall in pulse and respiratory rates; fall in blood pressure; increased stiffness of the tissues; loss of reflexes.

Temperature below 80°F (26°C): Life-threatening heart irregularities develop below this temperature; few individuals survive body temperatures lower than 75°F.

Since the above symptoms cannot be relied upon to indicate the severity of hypothermia (i.e., core temperature), it is essential to have a thermometer capable of reading from 75° to 105°F to determine the degree of body-heat loss that has occurred. (Thermometers that can measure low body temperature are available from Carolina Biological Products, P.O. Box 187, Gladstone, OR 97027; from Zeal G.H. Ltd., 8 Lombard St., London, S.W. 19, England; and from Dynamed--sec references.) Rectal temperatures are more accurate than oral, but technically more difficult and less esthetic.

The treatment of choice for mild hypothermia (core temperature 95°F or higher) is replacing wet with dry clothing, adding more clothes or other insulation, administering warm (and, desirably, sweetened) fluids, and candy, sugar, honey or similar carbohydrates. For moderate hypothermia (core temperature 90° to 94°F) provide heat as rapidly as possible without burning the victim. The torso (particularly the chest and neck) should be the first body area to be warmed. Any practical method of accomplishing rewarming is acceptable in the wilderness. One technique is to encase the cold patient in a "cocoon," composed of sleeping bags, clothes and any other material that will retain heat, with one or two other healthy, warm persons; skin-to-skin contact is desirable. Exhaling near the victim's nose and mouth to warm the air inspired by the cold person may be helpful. Alternatively, other sources of heat such as hot-water bottles, warm stones, or any other practical heat source may be utilized. Heat should be administered until shivering ceases, and both mental function and body temperature have returned to normal.

If hospitalization in the near future is impractical because of time-distance problems, the moderately cold patient who is conscious and at least partially cooperative may be treated by rapid rewarming, if materials are available. Water between 104° and 112°F (40° and 44°C) should be used; the torso is immersed in the water until shivering has stopped and mental function has substantially improved. The extremities should be left out of the tub until "core warming" has been achieved. The patient's head should be supported throughout the rewarming process by a third party.

It should be reemphasized that the critical factor for survival is the temperature of the central "core" area of the body. The torso should therefore always be the first part of the body to be warmed. Heat may be applied to the extremities immediately following rewarming of the core area. It is dangerous to warm the extremities if the central part of the body is not being heated!

Profound multiple metabolic abnormalities occur with severe hypothermia (body temperature under 90°F). This low a body temperature is a life-threatening emergency! Every effort should be made to transport the victim to a hospital intensive-care unit as soon as possible. If that is feasible within a reasonable time, available heat sources should be utilized to "stabilize" the core temperature while the patient is being transferred to an acute-care facility; aggressive rewarming is not advisable under these circumstances.

If the hospital is many hours or even days away, the severely hypothermic person is unlikely to survive that much delay. In this desperate situation, applying immediate heat to the victim is justified, utilizing any or all of the methods previously described.

Intravenous fluids, heated slightly above body temperature and administered by health-care professionals, are helpful and often life-saving. This sophisticated treatment, of course, is available only when a rescue team has reached the side of a hypothermic victim. Heated, moistened oxygen or air is also beneficial, and other systems, such as the use of a portable hypothermia blanket, for use in the field are available when trained personnel arrive. These modes of therapy may be continued in the ambulance or rescue helicopter on route to the hospital.

Lastly, it is most important to remember that very cold patients may appear dead but may revive when body temperature is normalized. *If the victim still appears lifeless after rewarming, resuscitative efforts may be discontinued.*

Immersion Hypothermia

Hyperventilation (overbreathing) occurs for 1-2 minutes after sudden immersion in cold water. The initial several breaths are huge involuntary gasps. The likelihood of aspiration of water is substantial under these circumstances. Even if the head is well above water, hyperventilation symptoms (lightheadedness, palpitation, air hunger, etc.) may occur. Breath-holding capacity in water under 60°F (15°C) is 15-25 seconds, approximately 1/3 normal. Therefore, a person suddenly immersed in cold water has a definitely increased risk of drowning. In addition, muscular dysfunction increases with the coldness of the water, lessening the ability to swim, climb onto a floating object, put on a life jacket or take other meaningful self-rescue actions.

Lethal heart stoppage may occur, particularly in the elderly, following sudden immersion in cold water. If the situation is controllable, cold water should be entered gradually to minimize this risk and to decrease the involuntary overbreathing response.

Very few victims of accidental immersion in cold water who are wearing an adequate life jacket die from drowning. Body cooling (immersion hypothermia) is a greater threat to their life. Therefore, if the risk of capsizing under cold-water conditions exists, all boaters should be well prepared to cope with both of these problems!

After 10-15 minutes of immersion in cold water, shivering becomes conspicuous and continues. After 15-20 minutes, body-core temperature begins to fall in spite of the shivering and resultant increase in metabolic rate. Shivering reaches a maximum when body temperature is between 93° and 95°F. At these body temperatures, changes in intellectual function, increased pulse, and increased urine production occur. Patients reaching a body temperature of 86°F (30°C) are usually semi-conscious, are likely to drown, and face the increasing probability of life-threatening heart irregularities as core temperature continues to fall.

The amount of body fat is a major determinant of the cooling rate in humans. Another significant factor is body size; large individuals cool more slowly than small ones. Children are at greatest risk for severe hypothermia. Women have more subcutaneous fat than men but are physically smaller, so in general cool at the same rate as men in cold water.

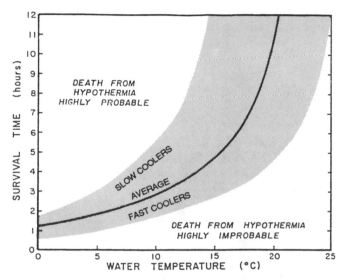

Predicted survival times for lightly clothed, nonexercising humans in cold water. The grey zone includes approximately ninety-five percent of the variation expected for adult and teenage humans. (From *Hypothermia, Frostbite and Other Cold Injuries*, by John S. Hayward. Reprinted by permission.)

In cold water, physical activity increases heat loss more than it increases heat production, so activities such as swimming accelerate core cooling. Physical activity in cold water should be avoided unless it is highly probable that the activity will get the individual at risk out of the water rapidly. The average individual is unlikely to be able to swim more than half a mile in water at 50°F (10°C), and lesser distances in colder water.

An effective personal-flotation device allows the person at risk to assume the heat-escape-lessening posture (HELP) or to huddle appropriately with others. Both maneuvers conserve body heat.

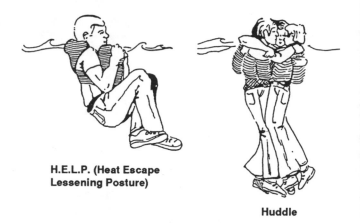

**H.E.L.P. (Heat Escape
Lessening Posture)**

Huddle

Methods for reducing the body surface area exposed to cold water

Heavy winter clothing will increase survival time, if one is immersed in cold water, about 35%.

A good personal flotation device should protect against hypothermia as well as drowning! It should be comfortable and should have good flotation characteristics, including face-up stability. It should also be highly visible, and should reduce convective and conductive heat loss to the water.

The more of the body that is out of the water, the less heat is lost. Therefore, getting on an overturned boat or raft is highly desirable, even if the wind is blowing. Put another way, the wind-chill factor is not as great a problem as the heat loss while immersed in cold water.

The will to live is important! Victims who panic are incapable of appropriate survival behavior as described above. Education before a immersion episode decreases the likelihood of panic behavior. Individuals running rivers, kayaking, or doing similar outdoor activities should be thoroughly instructed in immersion survival techniques prior to venturing on the water.

Mountain (altitude) Sickness

The density of the atmosphere decreases as altitude is gained. At high altitude, significantly less oxygen is available to the body, and lack of oxygen is the underlying cause of all five forms of altitude sickness. The severity of these problems differs widely among individuals, and to a lesser degree may vary in the same inidividual when exposed to the same altitude on different occasions.

High-altitude illness can be classified as follows:

1. Acute mountain sickness (AMS), manifested by headache, nausea, easy fatigability, vomiting, and a feeling of unwellness.
2. High-altitude pulmonary edema (HAPE), manifested by cough and progressive shortness of breath.
3. High-altitude cerebral edema (HACE), manifested by severe headache, loss of coordination (e.g., staggering gait), defective thinking, and progressive loss of consciousness.
4. Retinal hemorrhage (HARH), manifested by bleeding and swelling in the membranes lining the back of the eye;
5. Fluid retention of the face or extremities (peripheral

edema).

These five conditions often overlap, so that a given individual may show any combination of the five problems; they are part of a continuum, not separate afflictions.

(Edema means the accumulation of fluid. Cerebral means brain. Pulmonary means lung.)

It is apparent, then, that forms #2, #3, and #5 of high-altitude illness are due to abnormal fluid accumulations; it follows that the earliest sign of impending trouble is often the lack of the normal increase in urination at altitude.

All forms of high-altitude illness are better prevented than treated. The best prevention is slow ascent with gradual acclimatization to altitude!

A good working rule is: Do not ascend more than 1,000 vertical feet per day beginning at 9,000 feet. The altitude figures refer to where you sleep. Going temporarily high during the day may facilitate acclimatization, and seems to carry no hazard as long as one returns to the lower altitude to sleep. *The more these limits are exceeded, the greater the risk of developing mountain sickness.*

Acute mountain sickness *per se* is more miserable than serious. Pulmonary and cerebral edema are always serious conditions. The eye problems of HARH rarely cause major or permanent vision defects. Swelling of the face and legs is generally not a serious problem (though foot swelling may increase the risk of frostbite by making boots tight).

It is therefore most important that hikers, climbers and skiers who ascend to altitudes of 9,000 feet (2745 meters) or higher during their recreational pursuits be well aware of these conditions. Knowledge of the symptoms, signs and treatment measures may prevent severe illness or even death, which can occur in a relatively short time.

Since acute mountain sickness is not serious, its symptoms may be "toughed out." Further altitude gain should be avoided until symptoms improve, or preferably completely disappear. The drug Diamox may be used for both the prophylaxis and treatment of AMS. There are several prophylactic dosage schedules that are effective. Perhaps the most reasonable is to take 250 mg (one tablet) twice a day, starting the day of exposure to altitude, or alternatively at the first sign of suboptimal acclimatization, and continuing for 3 to 5 days while at altitude, or until the highest altitude contemplated is reached. The dosage for the treatment of AMS is 250 mg. twice a day. (The drug is a "fluid pill," and usually causes increased urination; a frequent side effect is numbness and tingling of the lips, fingers and toes.) For those whose only complaint is irregular breathing at night with associated insomnia or nocturnal headaches, a dose of one tablet at bedtime may be sufficient to substantially improve the problem. Symptomatic treatment with aspirin for headaches, Compazine (5 to 10 mg.) or a similar drug for nausea and vomiting, and rest for an appropriate period of time for high-altitude lassitude, may also be helpful.

Persons allergic to sulfa drugs should not consume Diamox.

Dexamethasone (a steroid, or cortisone-type drug) has recently been reported by most, but not all, investigators to be effective in both the prevention and the treatment of AMS. Prophylactic doses have been 4 mg. given orally (in contrast to the intravenous use in HACE) every 6 to 8 hours, generally starting 48 hours before ascent, and continuing for an additional 48 hours after altitude is reached. AMS and suspected withdrawal symptoms may occur if the drug is stopped abruptly; gradual tapering off may prove wise after further experience is gained. Prophylactic use should probably be reserved for those unable to tolerate Diamox.

The treatment dose is 8 mg. initially, with additional doses of 4 mg. given 6 and 12 hours after the initial dose. The drug may be used as emergency treatment for AMS to facilitate safe descent to a lower altitude. This drug and Diamox used together may produce better results than either medication alone. Both drugs may cause side effects, and therefore neither should be used for mild symptoms. Dexamethasone is more powerful than Diamox, but also more expensive and more likely to cause side effects; therefore, Diamox is best used to treat mild AMS symptoms, reserving dexamethasone for the severely ill.

HAPE is the abnormal accumulation of fluid within the air sacs of the lungs (alveoli) caused in some as yet unclear manner by the low oxygen content in the inspired air at high elevations. The incidence of HAPE is related to the highest altitude gained, the speed of ascent, and perhaps the age of the individual. Put another way, the higher one goes above sea level and the faster the speed of ascent, the greater the risk.

People under 21 may have a greater risk of developing HAPE than older people. The condition affects males more commonly than females.

Subclinical cases in which there are X-ray abnormalities, but no symptoms, occur perhaps 3 times as frequently as diagnosed cases with symptoms. Probably patients who have had the condition once are more likely to have the condition again on re-exposure to altitude than those who have been high previously without difficulty.

The mortality rate in clinically diagnosed cases varies between 1% and 10%. Signs and symptoms usually begin between the second and third days of overnight exposure to a higher altitude.

Fatigue and shortness of breath with exertion are the usual initial symptoms, along with a dry, persistent cough, especially apparent at night. Indeed, a cough not associated with the usual symptoms of a cold or upper respiratory infection must be considered a very suspicious and significant abnormality. Often there is a sense of chest oppression or a feeling that chest motion is difficult or restricted. A relatively good test in the field is to have the patient rest for approximately 30 minutes, and then check his resting pulse, which should be less than 110; his resting respiratory rate should be less than 20 under these conditions. Higher rates suggest early pulmonary edema (or other lung abnormalities, such as pneumonia). If a physician or nurse is present, checking for rales (moist crackles in the chest) in the lung bases is also helpful. This can be done by simply applying the ear against the chest wall if a stethoscope is not available. As the condition become progressively worse, the patient becomes short of breath at rest and develops a blue color to the skin, and the cough becomes wet, i.e., productive of phlegm. Obviously labored respiration develops, with bubbling noises in the chest. Shortness of breath becomes severe, even at total rest. These symptoms may progress inexorably until death occurs.

The treatment of choice is to descend at least 2,000 feet (610 meters) to a lower altitude immediately. Descent alone, particularly if done early in the course of the condition, may be completely curative without other treatment. Oxygen if available should be given at 2 to 4 liters per minute for 24 hours, if descent is not curative or is impractical. (The weight of this much oxygen is a formidable problem to all but major expedition parties.) Activity should be minimal until full recovery. There is considerable disagreement among authorities about drug therapy for HAPE, although all agree that digitalis is not effective. Although treatment with morphine is still somewhat controversial, the physician most experienced with the treatment of HAPE recommends morphine unreservedly, particularly in apprehensive patients with very rapid breathing rates. More controversial is the use of Lasix. Some experienced physicians feel that it is helpful in a dosage of 40-80 mg. given initially and 6 to 12 hours later; others feel that its use may be more harmful than beneficial. They think it may cause dehydration and abnormalities of the salts in the blood; certainly prolonged use of the drug is unwise if the patient develops a fluid-depleted appearance and complains of thirst.

All experts agree that prompt descent is the treatment of choice, and that other available therapy should be considered supplemental at best, or to be used only if immediate descent is impossible. (If the recently developed portable hyperbaric (Gamow) bag is available, its use offers an alternative to rapid descent if weather, darkness, or other conditions make going lower hazardous. This device weighs only 8 lbs., can be pressurized with a foot pump, does not require supplemental oxygen, and can be carried easily on expeditions.)

The lessened depth of respiration in normal sleep seems to accentuate HAPE (and AMS). Diamox therefore may provide some degree of protection for HAPE.

A number of common drugs are respiratory depressants to some degree. Therefore "sleeping pills," tranquilizers, cough suppressants, anti-pain drugs containing codeine, and anti-diarrheal preparations containing opiates (paregoric, Lomotil, etc.) should be avoided, particularly in the evening and during the night, since their use probably increases the risk of HAPE.

Nifedipine, a drug that dilates lung blood vessels, is of value in the treatment of HAPE. It is particularly useful when oxygen is not available, and/or descent is hazardous or impossible. The dose is 10 mg. orally every 6 hours of the standard strength capsules, or 30 mg. every 12 hours of the extended release (XL) tablets.

A simplistic explanation of HACE is that the accumulation of fluid in the brain, in some way due to lack of oxygen, causes it to swell. Since it is enclosed within a rigid skull, the brain cannot expand. Therefore, minor changes in brain volume result in substantial symptoms.

Common symptoms of HACE are severe headaches, inability to walk normally, hallucinations, double vision, emotional lability, disorganized thinking, projectile (forceful) vomiting, disorientation in time and place, confusion, progressive loss of consciousness, and ultimately death. The usual indications for an urgent descent are uncoordination (manifested by inability to walk in a straight line) and worsening of mental status.

Patients with the illness who return to a lower altitude early in the disease generally do well. With delayed evacuation, death is not uncommon. As with HAPE, the recommended management of HACE when it develops is rapid descent to a lower altitude at the earliest indication of significant symptoms! If descent is not possible, less effective (or adjunctive) therapy includes, in order of preference:

1. Oxygen is helpful at a flow rate of 2-4 liters per minute if somehow available, and if used early in the course of the illness.

2. Intravenous use of potent cortisone-like drugs in substantial doses (dexamethasone or betamethasone) shrinks the swollen brain temporarily; unfortunately the average climber will not have the drug or the expertise to use it. Even a physician climber is limited, since the drug must be protected from excessive heat and freezing, and sterile syringes, needles, etc. must be on hand (1 cc. or 4 mg. syrettes are available, but the usual initial dose is 10 mg., or 2.5 cc.). (Far more portable are 4 mg. oral tablets of these medications. However, tablets cannot be given to a person unable to swallow.)

3. If the patient is not dehydrated and blood pressure seems normal, a single dose of 80 mg. of Lasix orally (or an injectable dose of 40 mg.) may be helpful. Dehydration and low blood pressure are undesirable side effects of therapy, of particular concern if the victim is unable to take replacement fluids by mouth. (Professionals with appropriate equipment may combine Lasix given intravenously with supportive fluids also given by vein.)

Drug therapy is not a substitute for descent!

HARH may cause subjective visual defects; most people with this condition, however, are unaware of the problem. Nonetheless, 20-30% of people exposed to altitudes above 14,000 feet develop bleeding, which can only be seen by the use of a medical instrument called an ophthalmoscope. Most of the visual defects disappear with the passage of time; permanent partial loss of vision is unusual. Major visual abnormalities are best tested for with one eye closed, since the normal eye will often compensate for a defect in the involved eye. Significant vision loss (or the presence of objectively confirmed substantial hemorrhages) is justification for descent, or at the least for not gaining further altitude until subjective or objective improvement can be demonstrated.

Females (particularly premenstrually) are more susceptible to generalized water retention at high altitudes. This is more annoying than incapacitating usually; however, any accumulation of fluid (usually manifested by swelling of the face, hands, ankles or feet) calls for careful immediate assessment for the concomitant presence of early HAPE or HACE. (It is unwise to wear tight rings at high altitude.) Restriction of salt intake plus use of "fluid pills" (Lasix) will control the swelling. Premenstrual females should probably take a longer-than-average time for ascent to significant altitude, particularly if their previous experience shows excessive water retention during this phase of their monthly cycle.

Lastly and most importantly, if any combination of symptoms previously described suggestive of either cerebral or pulmonary edema develops, *GO DOWN AT ONCE,* even if emergency evacuation or traveling at night is necessary to accomplish the immediate descent. No summit or other mountain activity is worth dying for!

Drowning and Near-Drowning

Drowning is defined as submersion in water resulting in asphyxia and death while submerged, or within one day of the episode. Near-drowning is submersion of sufficient gravity to result in the victim being transported to the hospital, but not severe enough to result in death within 24 hours. Immersion syndrome is sudden death (reflexly induced heart stoppage) resulting from sudden contact with extremely cold water.

The usual sequence of events in drowning is an initial period of panic with a violent struggle and associated breath holding; if this is unsuccessful, the victim will swallow and/or inhale water. Vomiting is common. When fluid fills the lungs, death occurs rapidly.

There are complex physiological differences between fresh and salt water drowning, but these biochemical changes are usually not seen in near-drowning, since survivors have usually not inhaled much water, whether fresh or salty.

Most victims who are still breathing when removed from the water recover; nonetheless, *all individuals with significant submersion exposure should be hospitalized for observation for at least 24 hours.* Patients with lung disease are at greater risk from submersion than those with normal lungs.

If the circumstances of the water immersion could be associated with other injuries, as soon as breathing is restored, a complete examination for other abnormalities, such as a fractured neck or ruptured spleen, is essential.

The immediate treatment in the field for those still breathing is: Be sure the airway is clear, remove wet clothes and replace with dry ones to prevent hypothermia, and transport the patient to the nearest hospital as soon as possible. For those not breathing, mouth-to-mouth ventilation should begin immediately, if possible when the patient is still in the water. When out of the water, clear the airway and keep it clear thereafter. There is controversy as to whether the Heimlich Maneuver is of value in this regard. Lifting the patient transiently, by grasping about the abdomen (the pelvic bones provide hand-holds) so the head is down, may lead to drainage of fluids from the stomach and/or the lungs. Vomiting is common; if it occurs be prepared to prevent aspiration of vomitus. After the airway is clear, continue aggressive mouth-to-mouth ventilation. If there is no evidence of heart action, move to the CPR mode of alternating heart compressions with mouth-to-mouth ventilation. Try to keep the patient level (head neither down nor up) when CPR is being given. Continue for 1 hour or until futility is apparent.

For patients submerged for a substantial time in warm water who appear without respiration or heartbeat and who have widely dilated pupils, purple skin streaks, or generalized stiff muscles (rigor mortis), no resuscitation effort is indicated since the patient is clearly unsalvageable. If the patient is hypothermic, or the water in which he has been submerged is very cold, it is worthwhile to attempt resuscitation efforts, even if the victim appears dead, since occasionally functional survival will occur under these special circumstances. Hypothermic patients have survived with little or no residual brain damage after 40 minutes of submersion in very cold water.

The mammalian diving reflex may occur in children. This consists of heart slowing, blood shunting to the brain and closure of the airway. Under these circumstances, functional survival is possible for longer than usual after submersion, justifying more aggressive resuscitation efforts.

Alcohol is the chief drug implicated in submersion incidents. In one Australian study, over half of victims 26 and older who drowned had blood alcohol values at a level that would impair their ability to function. Swimmers, canyoneers, sea kayakers, and boaters should sharply limit alcohol intake before venturing into or upon the water.

Pneumonia

Pneumonia is a lung infection caused by several types of micro-organisms. Symptoms include chills, fever, cough, sharp chest pain when taking a deep breath or coughing, shortness of breath, and often the production of considerable amounts of yellow, green or rusty phlegm. The patient appears acutely ill.

Most pneumonias will respond to the administration of the antibiotics listed in the first-aid kit contents (cephradine or tetracycline). Mild pneumonias will respond to the lower dosage, but severe pneumonia should be treated with the dose recommended for severe infections. If improvement does not occur within 24 to 36 hours with one of the medications, switch to the other one, since the organism may be resistant to the first drug, but is unlikely to be resistant to both medications. It is important to differentiate pneumonia from HAPE and from blood clots in the lungs, since treatment of these three conditions is quite different. Even skilled physicians may have difficulty making a correct diagnosis. If in doubt, it may be wise to treat for all three conditions simultaneously. Certainly if a patient is being treated for pneumonia and fails to improve, management for the other two illnesses should be instituted.

Clots in Veins (phlebitis)

The increase in red blood count which occurs as part of the acclimatization to high altitude increases the "thickness" of the blood and thereby predisposes to clotting in the veins. Physical inactivity also predisposes to this condition since muscular exercise is the prime factor responsible for returning the blood to the heart from the extremities; inactivity allows the more viscous blood to "sludge" in the veins of the legs or lower abdomen and then clot.

Accordingly, climbers, particularly those doing expeditionary climbing at high altitude, when faced with long periods of inactivity due to inclement weather, should elevate their legs frequently and exercise all the leg muscles vigorously. In particular, the ankle joints should be forcibly moved through their full range of motion at least once an hour during any period of prolonged inactivity.

If clotting in the leg veins does occur, it will often be manifested in pain and/or swelling in one or both lower legs. The calf muscle is frequently tender if compressed. If another individual forcibly and sharply moves the toes of the involved leg toward the body, pain will be experienced in the calf of the leg. The danger of this condition is that a clot may break loose from the involved vein and lodge in the lung, causing a serious or occasionally fatal illness. If phlebitis does occur, the treatment thereof becomes a medical emergency which cannot be undertaken in the field, and the climb should be aborted immediately and the attention of a competent physician sought.

Lightning

Injuries from a lightning strike can range from mild to severe. A person hit by a major bolt appears dead, since both heart action and breathing cease; however, the chances of recovery are quite good if effective external heart compression and mouth-to-mouth artificial respiration are started immediately and continued as long as necessary. (Rescuers should realize that they too are at risk, since lightning does strike the same place twice.) Less severe, and fortunately completely reversible, injuries include burns, fractures and temporary paralysis. Eye and ear damage may occur, leading to permanent, partial or total blindness and deafness.

Although it is a terrifying experience, complete recovery is the expectation for those who are stunned but obviously alive after being struck by lightning.

By way of prevention, avoid summits, ridges, open flat meadows, solitary tall trees, wet marshy areas, and small caves or exposed overhangs when thunderstorms are nearby. Remove all metal from your person and immediate vicinity.

Drinking Water

A research study conducted in the summer of 1965 on high mountain water in the North Cascades indicated that many of the water sources commonly used by mountaineers are contaminated with bacteria originating in the stools of native animals, stock animals or human beings. Water from high mountain tarns and streams issuing directly from snow fields was generally safe to drink without treatment; all other high mountain water sources were generally contaminated. As a working rule, then, it behooves the climber to consider most water available to him as contaminated (particularly in the Third World), and to treat it appropriately.

Several methods of decontaminating water are available. Perhaps the simplest, but often not practical because of lack of fuel, is to strain the water and then heat it to a rolling boil. Since temperatures above 65°C kill all disease-causing bacteria, the effect of altitude on lowering the boiling point can be disregarded. (At sea level water boils at 100°C.) It is safe to drink after cooling. A pinch of salt per quart may improve the taste after boiling, as may pouring the water from one container to another.

If boiling is impractical, the water desirably should be strained through a clear cloth to remove any sediment or floating matter. Several chemical treatments may then be used.

1. Probably the easiest and most effective water purification method is to use tetraglycine hydroperiodide (Potable-Aqua;* Globaline), an iodine compound.

    These tablets lose effectiveness when exposed to air or moisture. It is important to recap the container tightly immediately after each tablet is removed; be sure that water does not contaminate the remaining tablets. Do not rely on iodine pills that have been air-exposed for a substantial time. The manufacturer recommends discarding the remaining tablets contained in an open bottle after one year even though it has been tightly stoppered. Unopened bottles should retain potency for about four years. Store the iodine tablets in the refrigerator between backcountry trips.

    Add one tablet per quart to clear water or two tablets per quart to discolored water. Wait until the tablet dissolves, shake well, and then allow a bit of treated water to contact the screw threads and cap. Wait 10 more minutes before using. (Note: follow the

---

*Available in many outdoor stores or from Wisconsin Pharmacal Co., P.O. Box 198, Jackson, WI 53037.

same procedure if using other chemical disinfectants.)

2.   Iodine is also available as a 2% tincture. Add 5 drops per quart of clear water or 10 drops per quart of cloudy water and let stand 10 minutes before using. One drop disinfects a standard size glass of water.

3.   Chlorine tablets (Halazone) are not as effective against certain disease-causing agents as iodine, but may be used if iodine is not available. Add two tablets per quart (four tablets if the water is cloudy or presumably heavily contaminated) and allow to stand for 30 minutes before drinking.

Be aware that chemical disinfection works slower if the water is cold (see **Giardiasis** below).

Any number of devices have been marketed over the past few years which are claimed to remove parasites such as *Giardia*, amoeba and bacteria from contaminated water. Most rely on a filtering system to remove infectious organisms; some also utilize chemicals to kill germs and parasites.

Few if any of these devices will filter out or kill viruses. The virus of greatest concern is the one causing infectious hepatitis (liver inflammation), a disease considerably more serious than giardiasis. Costs vary from a low of about $20 for the Pocket Purifier to as high as $725 for the Katadyn expedition water filter. Water production from many of these devices is slow and tedious. Although generally effective for the removal of bacteria and parasites (giardia and amoeba), some of the devices may not remove infectious agents from contaminated water totally. In addition, some may cease to be effective after they have been in use for some time, without the loss of protection being apparent to the user; in other words, some devices do not "fail safe."

There may well be special circumstances in which a device is the best way to deal with contaminated water; however, for the average hiker, backpacker or climber, a technique of proven effectiveness, such as boiling or use of iodine, is probably the best present solution for removing disease organisms from wilderness water supplies.

Materials frequently added to water bottles, such as Milkman and Wyler's drinks, should be put in the water container only after the iodine has done its work. If added sooner, the food materials may inactivate the iodine.

Giardiasis (Backpackers' Diarrhea)

Infections with the protozoan *Giardia lamblia* are a common cause of diarrhea in the Third World. Giardiasis has recently been recognized to be a not infrequent cause of diarrhea in the United States. The organism appears to be particularly prevalent in the water of mountainous regions throughout the world.

Clinically, bowel symptoms may be brief and self-limited; more commonly the disease presents with explosive, watery, foul-smelling bowel movements; associated symptoms are lack of appetite, nausea, gas and abdominal bloating. Chills and vomiting may occur. Stools are bulky and bloodless. If untreated, weight loss and malnutrition may eventually occur.

The diagnosis is made by identification of cysts in the stool, or by aspirating material from the upper part of the intestinal tract if bowel-movement examinations are negative and the disease is strongly suspected. A newer and probably more accurate test is to assess for the presence of a specific antigen (protein) present in the parasite (EIA test for Giardia specific antigen 65. Three drugs are currently available in the U.S. for treating giardiasis. These are quinacrine (Atabrine), metronidazole (Flagyl) and furazolidone (Furoxone). The Atabrine dose is 100 mg. three times a day; authorities recommend a minimum of 5 and a maximum of 10 days of treatment. Flagyl may be given as a single oral dose of 2.0 grams for 3 consecutive days, or 750 mg. 3 times a day for 5 days, or 250 mg. 3 times a day for 5 to 10 days. Higher doses and longer treatment times improve the cure rate. Furoxone is available in liquid form, and useful for treating small children. Infestations resistant to one drug usually will respond to another. Cure rates vary from 70-95%. Those who respond usually do so promptly and relatively dramatically. Therefore, if far from a laboratory, a therapeutic trial with Atabrine or Flagyl may well be justified for diarrhea that lasts over one week. (Alcohol should not be consumed while taking Flagyl.)

Giardiasis is most commonly acquired by drinking contaminated water containing the organism. Bringing water to a boil kills this parasite. Iodine in low concentrations also destroys *Giardia*, but the killing action is slower as the temperature of the water decreases. Therefore, the recommended contact time between iodine and water at a near-freezing temperature is considerably longer than the usually advised 10 minutes. Alternatively, higher doses of iodine can be used to decontaminate chilled water. Practically, since clear-cut research data is lacking, it would be best to boil near-freezing water. If that is impractical, a reasonable approach would be to treat very cold water for 30 minutes with standard doses of iodine, or for 15 minutes with double the usual dose (see the section on drinking water).

Diarrhea

Transient diarrhea in the U.S. is usually due to changes in food intake and/or established habit patterns. Since symptoms are self-limited, drug therapy is not indicated. The basic treatment of all diarrhea, regardless of cause, is the prompt replacement orally of the fluids and salts being lost from the colon. Therefore, the afflicted should drink soups and broths, fruit juices, pasteurized milk, and similar liquids rather than water alone; add table salt liberally to the liquids consumed when possible. Intake of liquids should exceed fluid losses by at least one quart in cool climates, and two quarts in hot areas.

In Asia, Africa, Mexico, and Central and South America, traveler's diarrhea affects 30-50% of people within two weeks after arrival. The most common causative organism produces benign, self-limited disease; less common bacteria and parasites can cause more serious illness.

The likelihood of developing traveler's diarrhea can be substantially decreased by prophylactic consumption of several medicines; these include doxycycline, Pepto-Bismol and trimethoprim/sulfamethaxazole; however, unless time is limited and the mission crucial, prophylactic therapy is not now recommended for most foreign travelers. If prophylaxis is elected, Pepto-Bismol is probably the drug of choice, using a dose of 2 tablets 4 times a day. Aspirin should not be taken while on Pepto-Bismol.

Using good judgment about where and what one eats, and treating persistent diarrhea if it develops, are probably the best ways of dealing with the problem. For mild illness without fever, an agent that acts nonspecifically, such as Bismuth subsalicylate (Pepto-Bismol) may be useful.

Tablets should be chewed or dissolved in the mouth. Adult dosage is 2 tablets every 30-60 minutes to a maximum of 8 doses in a 24-hour period. For more severe diarrhea, with or without fever, trimethoprim/sulfamethaxazole (trade names Bactrim-D.S., or Septra-D.S.) can be given twice a day for 3 days. An alternative medication is a quinolone (Cipro 500 mg. every 12 hours for 5-7 days). Symptoms resolve on average 30 hours after the beginning of treatment. Failure to respond to therapy suggests infection with unusual bacteria or an intestinal parasite (amoeba or *Giardia*); travelers with persistent post-treatment diarrhea should seek medical attention.

Imodium A-D 2 mg. caplets are available without prescription; 2 caplets may be taken initially after the first loose bowel movement; one caplet may be taken after each loose stool thereafter, up to 4 doses every 24 hours. Prescription drugs for the control of diarrhea include Lomotil (2 tablets 4 times a day), or codeine 30-60 mg. (one or 2 tablets) 4 times a day. These drugs usually relieve cramps and decrease the frequency of stools, but they do not kill the causative organisms; therefore, their use may prolong the illness. Consequently, use of these drugs should be reserved for more severe episodes (in conjunction with the specific therapy as detailed above) or circumstances where terrain and/or weather make frequent elimination impractical or hazardous.

Foreign Travel Advice

Individuals considering travel to other than Canada, New Zealand, Australia and Western Europe should contact their physician or local health department well in advance of departure for medical advice regarding AIDS, traveler's diarrhea, immunizations, and malaria prophylaxis. An excellent summary of recommendations can be found in the May 1, 1992 issue of the Medical Letter.

Appendicitis

This illness is a surgical emergency! Persons with suggestive symptoms should abort other activities and seek surgical consultation as soon as practical. The usual picture is of abdominal pain of increasing severity, eventually localizing in the right lower abdomen. Fever, nausea and vomiting, and lack of appetite are other findings. The abdomen is usually tender. Diagnosis can be difficult even for skilled physicians, since about 25% of cases do not show the usual findings listed above. If there will be a delay of over six hours in obtaining medical assistance, and the disease is suspected, it would be wise to take antibiotics until a surgeon can be consulted, since these drugs may slow the progress of the condition. (If vomiting occurs within 30 minutes after giving the antibiotics, readminister the medication on the assumption that most of the dose has been lost.)

Nausea and Vomiting

Being sick to the stomach and throwing up are symptoms of many illnesses, and not a diagnosable disease in and of themselves. The significance of the symptom and the severity of the vomiting depend on the nature of the underlying disease process. Vomiting without fever or abdominal pain is probably due to nonserious disorders, such as food intolerance or virus infection of the intestinal tract. Sometimes the act of vomiting resolves the problem by expelling the noxious material. Benign vomiting may be treated with drugs, such as Compazine, orally or rectally, as needed to control this unpleasant symptom. From 5 to 10 mg. of Compazine every 4 hours orally, or 25 mg. every 4 hours rectally, are appropriate doses. If vomiting occurs within a half hour of oral administration, re-give the dose.

On the other hand, if associated with fever and abdominal pain, vomiting may indicate a serious process requiring medical attention as soon as possible (see the section on appendicitis). Persistent vomiting causes problems of fluid loss. Even if there is no serious underlying process, the dehydration itself may mandate medical attention. Lastly, vomiting in an unconscious or semiconscious patient requires immediate action to prevent vomited material from entering the windpipe. Turn the patient on to his side or face down; lift the midportion of the body (the pelvic bones provide handholds) so that the chest is higher than the mouth until vomiting has ceased and all of the regurgitated material has been cleared from the back of the mouth, and the throat.

Snow Blindness

Excessive exposure to sunlight, associated with extensive travel on snow, ice or less commonly water or granite, may cause eye redness, spasm of the eyelids, defective vision and eye pain if the eyes are not protected from the excessive glare. There is a several-hour delay between overexposure to sunlight and the development of symptoms. Distress may be so substantial in severe cases as to cause almost total blindness temporarily. The use of eye goggles, or appropriately curved sun glasses, desirably with side masks, at times of substantial light exposure is an effective preventive. The lenses must effectively screen at least 90% of the harmful *ultraviolet* light, and therefore should be carefully selected with the assistance of a competent professional. Many cheap "over the counter" sun glasses do not screen the harmful light rays satisfactorily.

Symptoms are invariably bilateral; involvement of only one eye indicates some other sort of problem. Drugs that dilate the pupil help in relieving pain. Cyclogyl 1% is a useful medication for this purpose; one drop is instilled in each eye every 6 hours until symptoms abate. Expect a stinging sensation when Cyclogyl is instilled. Even if drugs are not used, increased eye protection with double goggles, a blindfold, etc., is mandatory as soon as possible after the onset of symptoms; it is particularly important to protect the eyes from further light damage if the pupil has been dilated with medicine. One climbing physician carries sterile eye patches, which he applies using scotch tape.

Cool moist compresses applied over closed eyelids, aspirin, and, if necessary, codeine may be utilized to provide pain relief. Local anesthetic ointments or drops, such as Pontacaine, will also relieve symptoms, but should be avoided since they delay healing of the delicate eye membranes. However, if vision for a time is necessary for survival, the hazards of temporary usage of Pontacaine may have to be accepted until a safe haven is reached. Topical steroids (cortisone-like eye ointments) shorten the duration of symptoms, and there is little risk in using these medicines for a short time (i.e., three days or less). Since the injury is physical, the risk of infection is minimal, and antibiotics locally or by mouth are probably not indicated. A pupillary dilator should not be used by an individual known to have an elevated eyeball pressure (glaucoma).

Fortunately, snow blindness rarely if ever causes any permanent loss of vision.

Sunburn

Prevention is clearly better than treatment!

Each 1,000-foot increment in altitude increases the intensity of sunburn-producing ultraviolet light by 4%. Fresh snow reflects 70-90% of ultraviolet light; reflection from water is variable, nearly 100% when the sun is directly overhead, but much less if the sun is lower in the sky. Reflected light may be especially damaging, because it often strikes the skin in normally unexposed, untanned and therefore unprotected areas, such as the roof of the mouth, under the chin, and inside the nose. No Caucasian individual has sufficient skin pigment to prevent sunburn on a bright day at altitude while on snow or ice.

Sunscreens have immeasurably improved over the past few years; they are available without prescription. The substantivity of a sunscreen is its ability to remain effective under the stress of prolonged exercise, sweating or swimming. The sun protection factor (SPF) is the ratio of the time required to produce redness through a sunscreen compared to the time required to produce the same degree of redness without the sunscreen. For example, if you sunburn in one-half hour without a sunscreen, you will burn to the same degree in 7½ hours with a properly applied SPF 15 preparation. For extremely sun-sensitive skins, or with intense exposure (summer climbing on snow or ice), a preparation with a SPF rating of 29 or higher (such as Pre-Sun 29) is advisable. Most people under standard conditions will do well with materials with ratings from 8 to 15. Trial-and-error selection of a preparation that protects your particular skin type and is aesthetically acceptable is suggested. (See the Medical

Letter, pages 61-63, June 17, 1988, for additional information.) The sunscreen should be applied to all exposed areas with sufficient frequency to be effective, and desirably should be applied an hour before sun exposure. Do not apply into or near the eyes. Wear sunglasses and a hat with a brim to protect the skin around the eyes. The wearing of protective clothing, such as gloves, hat and long-sleeved shirt, is an even more appropriate method of preventing sunburn.

Sunburn-preventing lip creams are now also available, such as RV PABA lipstick, made by the T.C. Elder Co.

Regular use of sunscreens also prevents aging changes of the skin, and lessens the likelihood of the eventual development of skin cancers. Adverse effects include the development of allergic reactions to the chemicals in the sunscreen.

Mild sunburn needs no treatment other than aspirin. More severe cases should be treated like a thermal burn with Vaseline, sterile gauze dressing and an elastic wrap, plus codeine if aspirin does not control the pain.

There is evidence that steroid (cortisone-like) drugs benefit the patient with acute sun-induced burns. The sooner after exposure these drugs are used, the more rapid is the response. The drug dose varies with the severity of the burn. Between 20 and 80 mg. of prednisone daily, preferably given as one dose in the morning, can be used. Prednisone is a potent medication, and supervision by a physician is highly desirable. If available, a steroid skin cream (Synalar 0.025%) may speed healing and reduce the discomfort of a moderate sunburn; apply thinly 4 times a day.

Several medications, including tetracycline,

predispose to abnormally severe sunburns in an occasional susceptible individual.

Thermal Burns

Burn severity depends on what amount of body area is involved, how deeply the skin is damaged, and what body areas have been injured. Burns of the crotch, feet, hands, armpits, face and neck are more difficult to manage, and always require medical attention.

Doctors call a mild or superficial burn a first-degree injury; examination findings are of skin redness. A moderate-depth burn (second-degree) causes blisters to form eventually. A burn that completely destroys the entire skin (third-degree) may look pale and white, or charred; since nerve endings are destroyed, less pain is felt in third-degree burn areas (margins where the burn is less deep may be quite painful). Even trained professionals have difficulty telling the depth of a burn immediately after the injury has occurred.

Two guidelines for determining the extent of the burn follow: (1) The rule of nines states that the head comprises 9%, the arms 9% each, the legs 18% each, the anterior trunk 18%, and the posterior trunk 18% of the total body surface area. (2) The palm area of an adult patient is approximately 1% of the total body surface area.

Extensive moderate or deep burns of more than 10% of the body surface are dire emergencies requiring immediate evacuation. Until evacuation can be achieved, keep the patient warm and, if he is not nauseated, give warm salty fluids by mouth to replace the body fluids lost from the burn area. Cold, moist dressings are more dangerous than useful for major burns.

For mild to moderate burns involving less than 10%

of the body, immerse the burned area in cold water for 2-5 minutes, if that can be accomplished within 15 minutes of the time of the injury. Pour cold water on the area if immersion is not possible. The sooner the burn is cooled, the better! Then remove clothing and jewelry from the area of injury. Cleanse the burned area as much as possible, ideally using sterile gauze, sterile water (iodine-treated or boiled and then cooled) and a liquid soap; if sterile material is not available, use the cleanest available cleansing agents. Following cleansing, apply sterile Telfa pads (if on hand) over the burned area. Another option is to apply sterile petroleum jelly (Vaseline) and cover the dressed area with either sterile Telfa pads or sterile gauze pads. (Under wilderness conditions, a dry sterile or clean dressing usually must suffice, although it will stick to the wound during later removal.) Cover whatever dressing is used with sterile (less desirably, clean) bulky material. Hold these materials in place with a snug bandage; an elastic bandage works well where it can be used. It should be applied in a manner that produces a moderate amount of pressure upon the burned area; care must be taken to avoid overcompression, which could compromise the circulation as swelling occurs. If circulation appears intact, leave the dressings in place until professional help is at hand.

If the patient must remain in the wilderness for a substantial time (24 hours or longer), and if there is reason to suspect that the burn has become infected (chills, fever, red streaks above the dressed area, lymph-gland enlargement in the groin or armpit, or visible pus at the burn site), the patient should be started on an antibiotic.

It is important to emphasize that creams, ointments, greases and other materials should not be applied directly onto the burned skin surface.

Substantial burns may be quite painful. Medications that relieve pain may be utilized to the degree necessary. Start with aspirin, Tylenol, or ibuprofen; add codeine to the degree necessary. If morphine is available, it may be used if the other drugs are not controlling the pain, provided there are no concomitant head injuries or breathing problems.

Baro-Otitis

Baro-otitis (damage to the ear drum due to rapid unequalized change in pressure between the outer and middle ear) occurs in individuals when allergy or infection causes blockage of the tube between the nose and middle ear.

It is rare that climbers ascend fast enough (save in a car) to have this difficulty; however, a rapid descent of 400-500 vertical feet while glissading could cause this problem. Symptoms include pain in the involved ear, hearing one's own voice more loudly than usual, and hearing external noises with diminished intensity. Prevention and treatment involve the use of a nasal decongestant (Teldrin), nose drops (Neo-Synephrine ¼ or ½%), and maneuvers designed to open the tube between the nose and ear, such as yawning and swallowing; even more effective is taking a deep breath, closing the mouth, holding the nose and "bearing down," swallowing simultaneously. If these maneuvers are ineffective and symptoms persists, the problem should be treated by an ear, nose and throat specialist.

Snakebite

Controversy regarding the preferred treatment for

snakebite continues. Authorities with varied professional backgrounds differ in their recommendations for management. The following procedures for the treatment of crotalid (rattlesnake, copperhead and moccasin) bites represent a current consensus with regard to management in the field. Coral-snake bites and bites of venomous snakes found outside of the United States are beyond the scope of this book.

Rattlesnakes range widely in the United States, often to high elevations in the Sierra Nevada and the Rocky Mountains. Moccasins (cottonmouths) are semi-aquatic snakes found in the southeastern United States. Copperheads occur in the eastern and southern states. Reasonable alertness will usually avoid close encounters, since these reptiles will make an effort, unless surprised or attacked, to avoid hikers and climbers. For obvious reasons, the terrain should be scrutinized carefully when hiking or climbing in areas known to harbor venomous snakes. Another obvious precaution is to wear high boots and long pants when in rattlesnake country.

Snake-venom poisoning is an emergency! Effective treatment must be instituted immediately following a bite, and should include measures to (1) retard absorption of the venom; (2) remove as much venom as possible from the wound; (3) neutralize the venom; and (4) prevent complications, including a secondary infection.

Following a snake bite, the first step is to identify the biting reptile to determine whether it is a poisonous snake. Use caution, since a snake that has bitten once may certainly bite again. Ideally, a companion of the bitten person should make this assessment.

Next, look at the wound to see if fang puncture marks are present. If there are no fang holes, significant poisoning is unlikely and the wound should simply be washed with soap and water, dressed, and observed over the next hour.

If the snake is venomous, and fang marks are present, and if a Sawyer First Aid Extractor is available, suction should immediately be applied over the fang punctures, using this device. The sooner it is applied, the more venom can be removed from the wounds before the poison spreads to the rest of the body. The power pumping action provided by the extractor is sufficient to remove venom without the need of the incisions previously required to facilitate less effective methods of suction. Follow the instructions provided with the kit, except for the recommendation of leaving the apparatus on for "up to 3 minutes for snake bites." After applying the device, Dr. Russell recommends leaving it on for 10 minutes or so, removing it to empty the blood, venom, and other fluids removed from the bite, and then reapplying it. This process is repeated for up to 40 minutes from the time of original application. (Caution: the pump should not be used on the eyelid or genital areas.) Sawyer kits may be obtained from REI, Sumner, WA 98352-0001 or from Dynamed; the price of the device is $14-$15 presently.

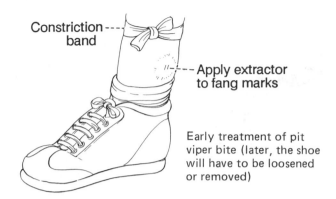

Constriction band

Apply extractor to fang marks

Early treatment of pit viper bite (later, the shoe will have to be loosened or removed)

After applying the extractor, begin making arrangements for transportation of the patient to the nearest hospital. Seventy-five percent of those bitten by a pit viper will develop significant problems.

Early symptoms of envenomation are burning pain, swelling at the site of the bite, weakness, nausea and tingling (pins-and-needles) sensations. Lack of any symptoms (other than minor discomfort at the site of the injury) 30 minutes after being struck is strong evidence that serious poisoning has not occurred. If symptoms develop, have the patient lie down if feasible, and limit use of the bitten area. Provide supportive care and encouragement. Remove all potentially constrictive devices, such as rings and bracelets, before swelling makes removal impossible. Proceed with evacuation of the envenomed person to the hospital as soon as possible. Do *not* use incision and suction, even if a Sawyer device is not available. Use of a constriction band, as shown in the above diagram, is elective. If a hospital is nearby, it is best not applied. If hospitalization will not be possible for several hours or longer, the band may be of some value, assuming the bite is on an extremity. The band should be about an inch wide. It is applied 2-4 inches toward the body from the fang marks. The band should be snug, but not tight enough to block the blood circulation. If progressive swelling develops, loosen the band if it becomes too tight, and move it several inches closer to the torso. The device should not be used longer than 2-3 hours. An elastic bandage is an alternative to the constriction band. It should be applied snugly, but not tightly enough to block arterial or venous circulation. Begin the application about 6 inches from the bite, and wrap toward the fang marks, stopping about 2 inches away from the wound. The purpose of these devices is to occlude the flow of venom through the tissues (via the lymphatics).

Antivenin is the definitive treatment of choice in the hospital setting. It can be a dangerous medication in sensitized persons, and should never be administered to a patient who has a history of allergy to horse serum or who has previously been treated with horse serum, save in the intensive-care unit of a hospital. Antivenin should be given only by a health-care professional; skin tests to exclude allergy are mandatory before administration. The sooner this material is given after the bite, the more effective it is, so time is of the essence in obtaining definitive treatment.

Whether antivenin should be utilized in the field by a paramedic or a physician is controversial; if severe symptoms of poisoning are developing rapidly and hospitalization is impossible in the foreseeable future, the benefits of antivenin administration may outweigh the risks. The professional at the scene must make this difficult decision.

Antivenin (Crotalidae) Polyvalent is made by the

Wyeth Company and supplied in containers measuring roughly 6 x 2½ x 1½ inches. The material is expensive. The minimal effective dose is 5 vials; more severe envenomations require 10-15 vials. Information on storage, reconstitution, and administration is provided in a brochure with each container. Antivenin gradually becomes inactivated as time passes, and must be discarded about 5 years after it has been manufactured. It should be stored in a cool place. Most hospitals in snakebite areas stock this material.

If hospitalization will be delayed 24-48 hours, and there is severe tissue involvement, consideration should be given to administering antibiotics. Tylenol and, if necessary, codeine may be used to control pain. Aspirin is a less desirable drug since it may worsen bleeding complications induced by the toxic properties of the snake venom.

(In July 1986, high-voltage electrical shocks were reported as being effective in the treatment of snakebite. Confirmation of effectiveness by other experienced physicians has not yet appeared. It is therefore most unlikely that this form of treatment is of value.)

Insects

In some persons, numerous bites cause allergic reactions with general sickness and considerable pain. Antihistamines may control the allergic reaction, and aspirin or codeine the pain. Severe itching is relieved by local application of a warm, moist cloth. Anyone known to be highly sensitive to insect bites or stings should be evaluated and perhaps desensitized in advance of the climbing season by a competent allergist and/or should carry a kit containing special medications for emergency treatment of acute allergic reactions (available on prescription). Epinephrine by injection is the treatment of choice for severe or life-threatening reactions following insect stings. This material is included in the Hollister-Stier AnaKit (anaphylaxis emergency treatment kit). The physician prescribing the kit should instruct those at risk in the use of the kit medications, since epinephrine administration is not simple or without risk.

If the sting is by a bee, the stinger should be removed promptly and gently. Do not apply mud or foreign materials. Aspirin applied topically has been reported to relieve discomfort after insect stings. Crush an aspirin tablet. Moisten the sting area. Apply the aspirin powder. Reapply moisture and medication as needed to control pain. Alternatively, the Sawyer Extractor, if applied immediately, may be of value in reducing the severity of insect stings (see the snakebite section).

Insect Repellents

The July 19, 1985 edition of the Medical Letter contains a list of the ingredients of a number of commonly used insect repellents. The most effective topical insect repellent is N,N diethyl-meta-toluamide, commonly called DEET. Topical repellents are usually effective for up to several hours, but can be removed from the skin sooner by wiping, sweating, or exposure to water. They must be reapplied under those circumstances to maintain effectiveness. If both an insect repellent and a sunscreen are being used simultaneously, the sunscreen should be applied first and allowed to dry, and then the insect repellent should be applied.

The material should be kept out of the eyes and

mouth, and removed from hands and fingers before handling food. Other directions on the label should be carefully followed. These compounds repel mosquitoes satisfactorily, are less effective against biting gnats, ticks, and chiggers, arc of little value against biting flies, and are ineffective against stinging insects, such as yellow jackets. Repellents containing DEET can cause allergic and toxic problems, including seizures; children are at greater risk for DEET toxicity than adults. Therefore, prolonged usage or excessive application of DEET repellents is inadvisable, since the long-term effects of DEET are unknown. Considering these facts, it is probably better to slap occasionally than to use these compounds. Usage should be reserved for when the bugs are intolerable, or when bites may cause serious illness, such as malaria or Lyme disease.

Commonly available repellents include 6-12, Off, Cutter's, Jungle Juice, and Muskol. The higher the concentration of DEET, the more effective the repellent, but the greater the likelihood of a toxic reaction.

Repellents containing tetrahydro-2-furaldehyde (R-11) were withdrawn from the market because of toxicity in 1989; anyone having a leftover supply containing this chemical should discard it. Currently available preparations do not contain this chemical.

A second approach to controlling insects is to wear protective clothing treated with permethrin. The simultaneous use of both DEET and permethrin is more effective than either used alone. Permethrin is available in most states, where it is sold in garden or sports stores as Duranon Tick Repellent. Contact Coulston International Corporation at P.O. Box 30, Easton, PA 18044 if you are not able to locate a local supplier.

The material is applied *to clothing only, not to skin!*

It kills ticks, chiggers and mosquitos on contact, rather than only repelling them. A one-minute application of the pressurized spray is adequate, applied before donning the clothing. For ticks, application to access areas (pant legs, sleeves and collars) is particularly important. No significant side effects of permethrin have been reported to date.

Ticks

Ticks are a potential hazard to climbers because they transmit certain illnesses. Repellents containing DEET offer protection against tick infestation if applied before exposure around all clothing openings. In addition, climbers in tick-infested areas should carefully examine their bodies for ticks at least once a day. Ticks that are found should be removed immediately.

Ticks may not attach themselves for hours after contact, and in this state can be easily removed. Once they have attached themselves, which is usually painless to the victim, removal is much more difficult. No simple, highly effective method of causing the tick to detach itself is known. Probably the best method is to grasp the animal with tweezers as close as possible to the point of attachment and remove by applying gentle traction; it is desirable, but not always possible, to remove the mouth parts with the rest of the tick. Every effort should be made to avoid crushing the tick and contaminating the bite site with crushed tick material. The wound should then be washed with soap and water and a bandaid applied.

If available, a recently developed instrument called "The Tick Solution" may be more effective than tweezers for removing the tick. Follow the directions on the back of the Tick Solution package, available from Instruments of

Sweden (134 Davenport Drive, Stamford, CT 06902, or from REI), approximate retail cost $11.50.

Tick bites can cause generalized muscular weakness known as "tick paralysis." Any unexplained weakness calls for careful search for, and removal of, ticks.

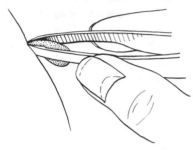

Removal of engorged tick with tweezers or forceps

In many areas of the U.S. (especially Montana, Oklahoma, Missouri, and the Carolinas) ticks can transmit the germs causing Rocky Mountain spotted fever, an illness characterized initially by fever, headache, sensitivity to bright light, and muscle aches. On the third to fourth day of fever, a pink rash usually appears. If not treated promptly with antibiotics (tetracycline), this disease may be lethal. Individuals with these findings and with known or suspected tick contact should obtain professional assistance as soon as possible.

Lyme disease is a recently recognized, widespread, tick-borne inflammatory illness. In the U.S., areas of high risk are in the Northeast, in the upper Midwest, and in California, southern Oregon, and western Nevada. Most cases develop between May 1 and November 30. The first abnormality is usually an expanding circular red rash, which occurs at the location where the tick had attached itself. Flu-like symptoms often develop shortly after the rash appears. Weeks to months later, serious heart, joint, and nervous system abnormalities may develop. The deer tick carries the bacteria that cause the disease. This tick, prior to engorgement, is very small (about the size of the dot above an i), and requires a very careful inspection to be seen before it has attached itself. Imbedded ticks should be removed immediately on discovery. Patients treated in the early stages of the disease with appropriate antibiotics usually recover promptly and completely. Anyone who has been in a high risk area who develops the typical rash should immediately see a physician.

A raised lump may develop at the site of a tick bite, and persist for a substantial time. These tick granulomas, if subjected to microscopic examination, may be erroneously diagnosed as a lymph-node cancer.

Animal Bites

The primary dangers from animal bites are infection in the wound and the possibility of rabies. Any bite should be washed thoroughly with soap and water and a sterile dressing applied.

Any mammal may carry rabies. If possible without hazard, the animal inflicting the bite should be captured or killed without damaging its head, so that the brain of the animal can be tested for rabies. Anti-rabies treatment of those bitten should start within 24 hours after the bite; time is of the essence and professional care should be sought immediately.

Bites of wild animals, particularly bats, skunks, foxes and raccoons, are especially suspect.

Plague

Wild rodents harbor the bacteria causing this disease. Fleas which have previously bitten an infected animal transmit the disease to man. Therefore, avoid ill or dead rats, mice and ground squirrels. Symptoms are high fever, prostration, muscle aching, and lymph-node swelling. Medical assistance should be sought immediately. If professional evaluation cannot be obtained within a few hours, and if this disease is strongly suspected, tetracycline should be administered.

Blisters

Blisters are caused by friction between the skin of the feet or ankles and poorly fitting boots, wrinkled or lumpy socks, or foreign bodies within the boot. Sweating is also probably a factor, since blisters occur more commonly when the weather is hot. To prevent blister formation, at the first sensation of foot discomfort take off the shoe, remove any foreign bodies, and straighten any wrinkles in the socks. If there are no obvious problems, apply a patch of Molefoam or Adhesive Foam (both made by Dr. Scholl's; both are equally useful) over the "hot spot;" the skin must be dry, or the material will not adhere. Be careful not to dislodge the patch when replacing the socks

If prior experience with a particular set of boots has indicated that hot spots or blisters inevitably develop in certain areas, it is wise to apply the protective material to those areas when the boots are first put on at the beginning of the hike or climb.

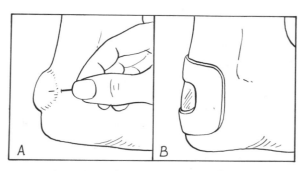

A method of managing a large blister

Small blisters should not be opened. Large blisters, or blisters obviously about to "pop," should have the fluid removed. Wash the area with soap and water. Sterilize the tip of a needle in a match flame, insert the needle tip in normal skin just beyond the edge of the blister, and pass it into the fluid-filled sac. Withdraw the needle and gently press out the fluid. Do not break the skin if at all possible. When all the fluid has been removed, cut out a patch of Molefoam substantially larger than the involved area. Cut a hole out of the center slightly larger than the blister and apply the Molefoam surrounding the blister. This will prevent further pressure or friction, and should protect the blister until the hike or climb has been completed.

If the skin over the blister has already broken, the resulting open wound should be treated with careful washing and application of a sterile dressing. If any evidence of a significant infection is present or develops, the use of an antibiotic is advisable. If further walking is necessary, it is well to protect the area with cut-out patches of Molefoam during the day. Sterile dressings, desirably of Telfa, which will not stick to the wound, should be applied when camp is reached and no more significant walking is necessary until the next day.

To remove Molefoam, wet the material; it can be taken off easily after a few minutes.

An alternative approach is to also use Spenco Second Skin for treating denuded blisters. After applying the Molefoam pad as shown in diagram B above, place the Second Skin over the raw area not covered by the Molefoam, and apply the Spenco adhesive knit to the Molefoam to hold the Second Skin in place. After the active walking day is over, the Second Skin is gently removed to permit cleansing of the area, and to allow the open area to dry. Telfa is then applied and left in place overnight. The following morning, before leaving camp, the above procedures are again followed.

Headaches

Save for mountain sickness, the causes of headache in the mountains are essentially the causes of headache in the normal environment. Treatment appropriate at home is effective in the mountains, aspirin being, in general, the drug of choice. Massage to the neck and relaxation of the neck muscles is often most helpful. The use of sun glasses to prevent eye strain from glare is also a preventive.

Muscular Cramps

Cramps in the legs during or after a long, strenuous day, particularly early in the season, are not unusual and sometimes may be disabling. These painful muscular contractions can often be prevented by a program of proper conditioning prior to intensive physical activity. Hikers and climbers who sweat profusely and replace sweat losses with water but inadequate salt may experience excruciating muscle cramps. These cramps are preventable by replacement of sweat losses with water or other fluids containing 2-3 gms. (½ tsp.) of salt per liter of water; indeed merely increasing dietary salt intake is often sufficient to prevent the problem from developing. Immediate stretching of the involved muscle, painful as this may be, may abort a cramp. If a full-blown cramp occurs, gentle massage of the involved area by another member of the party may be helpful. Adequate rest stops may also prevent the development of cramps.

Post Trauma Stress Syndrome (PTSS)

(A syndrome is a group of symptoms and physical findings that occur together, and characterize a particular abnormality.)

PTSS is an identifiable behavior pattern associated with the emotional stress of being involved in a threatened or actual death and dying situation. These psychological problems may follow exposure to a horrifying situation, either as a victim or as a rescuer. Symptoms may be severe, prolonged and disabling, and may include intrusive memories, flashbacks, anxiety, irritability, sleep problems (including nightmares), and inability to perform the usual tasks of daily living. Anyone involved in a gory disaster should feel free to discuss his feelings with others in the party during the evacuation process. Debriefing with a mental-health professional soon after the event may lessen the likelihood of PTSS, or ameliorate its severity.

Miscellaneous Outdoor Problems

Fishhook Wounds
Push barbed end out through the skin; clip off barb with pliers or clippers, then remove shaft of hook.

Splinters
Wash area thoroughly. Sterilize needle or tweezer tips in flame; pry out or push up and grasp splinter and remove; promote bleeding, rewash; dress with bandaid.

Fainting
If patient has not yet fallen, assist him rapidly to lie flat. If he has collapsed in a head-high position, lay him flat. Raise both legs 45°; recovery in 1-2 minutes will occur. Keep flat 10-15 minutes; resume erect position slowly.

Convulsions
Protect patient and team from hazards of terrain. Place a thick cloth between the teeth to prevent tongue biting. Unconsciousness, lethargy, confusion and poor judgment are common for several hours after a seizure. Give anti-epileptic medication as soon as patient can swallow (victim's own or 3-4 phenobarbital tablets).

Foreign bodies in the eye
1st—Pull upper lid over lower; move eye gently in all four directions; repeat 1-2 times, particularly after tear production is copious;
2nd—Have companion inspect eye; remove object gently with corner of handkerchief;
3rd—If object cannot be seen or removed easily, patch eye and seek a physician.

Boils, etc.
Hot pack as frequently as possible; when pus is visible, wash well and puncture one or more times with needle or knife tip sterilized in flame immediately beforehand;

drainage is contagious; burn dressings; wash hands.

Poison ivy (oak; sumac)
Successful strategies for lessening the risk of skin rash include: (1) Avoidance—learn to recognize the offending plants; (2) wear protective clothing and apply barrier preparations before exposure and every 4-6 hours thereafter; barrier creams include Stokogard Outdoor Cream, Ivy Shield, and Ivy Block. (3) Decontaminate during the day after known exposure with liberal use of water, and reapply barrier cream. (4) At the end of the day, apply an organic solvent such as isopropyl alcohol, followed by a water rinse. (5) Dispose of contaminated clothing and equipment so that the irritating chemical is not carried into the car, workplace or home.
Treatment: If contact was recent, rinse symptomatic areas copiously with body-temperature water as soon as possible to remove the irritating chemicals. Antihistamines (Teldrin 12 mg. every 12 hours) may be helpful. Cool, moist compresses relieve distress, and may be repeatedly applied. The most effective therapy is the administration of corticosteroid (cortisone-like) medications. Prednisone 40-60 mg. daily in 2-3 divided doses given by mouth is preferred initial therapy; dosage is tapered over the next 10-14 days. Steroid skin creams can also be applied directly to affected skin areas every 4-6 hours as solo therapy for mild cases, or as adjunctive care for severe inflammation; many brands are available (Diprosone; Diprolene; Syndar). Less potent creams should be used on the face and genital areas (hydrocortisone 1%).

Nosebleed
Ninety-five percent of nosebleeds can be stopped by

compressing the soft portion of the nose immediately below the bone between the thumb and the index finger and maintaining this pressure for ten minutes. Manipulation, picking and nose blowing should be avoided for 48 hours after the nosebleed stops.

Poisoning

Remove unabsorbed poison without delay. Induce vomiting by gagging with finger (unless victim is unconscious or has swallowed corrosive material). Identify poison if possible. If laxative available, induce diarrhea. Keep patient quiet, lying down and warm. Obtain medical assistance as rapidly as possible, particularly if victim is unconscious.

Heat Exhaustion

This problem may occur in conjunction with strenuous exertion in a hot environment. People engaged in strenuous exercise during hot weather should drink fluids containing salts (electrolytes) frequently, and perhaps apply water if available to the skin and clothing to assist with body cooling. Heat exhaustion is usually associated with failure to replace by mouth the substantial water (and salt) losses of profuse sweating. Faintness, malaise, palpitation, nausea, weakness, headache and muscle cramps are common symptoms.

The condition is rarely serious, and is best managed by lying down for a while in a cool place. Drinking 1-2 liters of cool water to which a small amount of salt (½ tsp. of table salt or two one-gram salt tablets per liter) has been added improves symptoms. Sprinkling water over the victim and then fanning to enhance evaporation is also helpful. Medical Letter consultants do not recommend salt and sugar solutions, such as Gatorade.

Heat Stroke
This may occur under the same environmental conditions
as heat exhaustion, but is much more serious. Body-
temperature control is lost due to the production of more
body heat than can be dissipated.

Symptoms include subjective sense of warmth,
confusion, staggering, headache and eventual coma. In
most cases, sweating is reduced or absent. Body
temperature is very high (105° to 106° F). This condition
is a medical emergency! Body temperature must be
lowered immediately. Immerse the patient in a cold stream
or lake, or apply cold water or snow compresses until body
temperature falls to near normal. Place the patient in a
cool, shady location during and following the cooling
treatment. Monitor body temperature frequently until
consistently normal.

Toothache
If available, instill oil of cloves in the cavity. If
unavailable, use aspirin and codeine for pain control until
a dentist can be consulted.

The Mountaineering First Aid Kit

All mountaineers and outdoorsmen venturing into
wilderness or remote areas must carry a first-aid kit and
must know how to use it. The following ingredients are
suggested as basic for the kit carried by individuals.

Medical Supplies
    1.   3-inch elastic bandage.
    2.   Bandaids, several sizes and at least three of

each.
3. Butterfly laceration dressings—at least 3—commercially available from Johnson & Johnson or can be made from adhesive tape.
4. Sterile 3 x 3-inch gauze squares—at least 3.
5. Razor blade (Schick is best) or bandage scissors.
6. Safety pins—several sizes.
7. Sunscreens (see section on sunburn).
8. Small cake of soap (or small 35 mm film can of soap powder).
9. In snake areas, snake-bite kit (Sawyer Extractor).
10. Needle (and thread).
11. Tweezers.
12. Mole*foam* (for blisters).
13. Talcum powder (in 35 mm film can).
14. Insect repellents.
15. Rubber gloves.

Drugs and directions for use

Adult dosages given; decrease dose for body weight under 100 lbs. and increase for body weight over 225 lbs.

Many drugs in standard use are inadvisable during pregnancy. It is wise to check for drug allergy before giving any medication.

1. Burns—Small tube of sterile Vaseline. After applying cold water (if promptly available), apply directly to the burn, then cover with sterile gauze and wrap firmly with ACE bandage. Use aspirin or, if necessary, codeine for pain control.
2. Snow blindness—1% hydrocortisone eye

ointment.* Have patient look up; pull lower lid down and fill cavity with ointment. Apply very dark goggle or preferably bandage the eyes after the medication is instilled.

3.   Mild pain—aspirin 0.3 grams #12. Two every 4 hours as needed to relieve pain (headache, muscular aches, etc.)

4.   More severe pain—codeine 30 mg. #6.* One-two every 4 hours (with 2 aspirin) to relieve more severe pain.

5.   Exhaustion—Dexedrine 5 mg. #2.* One every 4 hours. Dexadrine should be used only in survival situations where exhaustion may be life-threatening and where safety is available within a few hours of consumption of the stimulant medication. (This drug is not now legally available in some states.)

6.   Indigestion—One or two antacid tablets, repeated every 2-4 hours as needed (Alkets, Titralac, Tums, etc.). Nausea or vomiting—Compazine 5 mg. #4.* One (rarely two) every 4 hours.

7.   Diarrhea—Imodium A-D caplets #8 (alternatively Lomotil or codeine); see section on diarrhea for doses.

8.   Infections—Cephradine (a cephalosporin) 500 mg. #10*; one capsule every 12 hours for skin, soft tissue, and mild respiratory-tract infections; for urinary-tract infections, pneumonia, and severe infections, take one capsule every 6 hours. If allergic to cephalosporins, substitute tetracycline 250 mgs. #8. Mild infections—one capsule before

meals and at bedtime (do not take with milk or antacids); severe infections—one capsule every 3 to 4 hours day and night. (Note: antibiotic potency deteriorates with time; ask the pharmacist, when filling the prescription, to indicate the replacement date on the label.) Pregnant females and young children should not use tetracycline.

9. Heat, vigorous exercise, and profuse perspiration—salt tablets 1 gm. #10. Two tablets with each quart of water consumed under the above conditions. Tablets may cause stomach irritation if swallowed whole; dissolving the tablet in the liquid to be consumed is wise. One-half teaspoon of table salt is equally effective but less convenient. Salt should never be taken without adequate free water in the above proportions.

10. Allergies (hives, hay fever, etc.)—Teldrin spansules 12 mg. #4.* One capsule every 12 hours (makes occasional person torpid).

11. Dramamine 50 mg. #10—One 4 times a day to prevent or relieve motion sickness.

12. Ibuprofen (Advil, Nuprin) 0.2 grams #20. Two tablets 4 times a day to relieve inflammatory joint conditions such as tendinitis and bursitis. This drug is also a nonspecific pain reliever, and can be used to control other discomforts, such as headache and menstrual cramps.

13. "Sleeping pills"—Halcion 0.125 mg. #6*. One-half to one tablet at bedtime as needed to promote sleep. There is no such thing as a completely safe "sleeping pill;" all such

medication should be used with caution, particularly at altitude. Sedation and/or impairment in coordination the following day can occur with the use of any drugs of this type. Continued use may cause progressively increasing side effects. In addition, all of these drugs become progressively less effective if taken regularly. There is suggestive evidence that these drugs may increase the likelihood of high-altitude pulmonary edema if taken while at high altitude. (Over 10,000 feet, Diamox is probably both safer and equally effective for promoting sleep.) Nonetheless, insomnia can be a real problem for the climber, perhaps justifying intermittent short-term usage judiciously. People vary substantially in their susceptibility to sedative medications. It is therefore wise to start with a low dose and repeat in one hour if necessary (or to pre-determine the effective dose for each individual).

14.   Neosporin ophthalmic ointment*—for treatment of eye and superficial skin infections (instill in eye as per #2 above; place on infected area and cover with sterile dressing).

15.   If going to high altitude, carry Diamox 250 mg. #10; consider bringing nifedipine, Lasix, and dexamethasone; for directions, see the section on mountain sickness.

16.   Prednisone* 5 mg. tablets #10 and/or Synalar* skin cream 0.025% for treatment of severe sunburn and severe skin eruptions secondary to exposure to poison ivy, oak, or sumac.

17   Bactrim or Septra DS #6—One tablet twice a
        day to control traveler's diarrhea. If allergic to
        sulfa, substitute Cipro.
18.   Any medications necessary to treat the
        climber's individual medical problems, as per
        personal physician's instructions.

**The following additional material should be available in
the climbing party.**

1.   Plastic air splints (one full leg and one full
        arm size and/or a SAM splint).
2.   Hemostat (clamp).
3.   Arm sling (or shoulder immobilizer).
4.   Morphine—15 mg. (Tubex) #2.* Inject under
        skin to relieve severe pain every three to four
        hours. (Use with caution at high altitudes
        since it tends to depress respiration.)
        Morphine should not be used if there is a
        significant brain injury.
5.   Medium-sized adult oral airway (for head
        injuries; mouth-to-mouth resuscitation).
6.   Dexamethasone 4 mg. tablets #10 (if going
        above 10,000 feet overnight).
7.   Betadine (see comments in Wounds section).

THE KIT: A leather or plastic container is best; metal
containers are poor because of rust. Replace contents
regularly as used. All capsules deteriorate in heat—store in

---

*Available on physician's prescription only; it is understood that
medications available by prescription only will not be used by the
climber in self-treatment when professional attention is
available. In other words, don't take these drugs except in a
mountaineering emergency.

a cool place.

(# indicates number of items to be carried; in many cases, this is an inadequate amount for a full course of treatment, but will suffice until outside help arrives or until the climbing group can pool the resources of their combined first-aid kits.)

Finally, include this book for reference in your wilderness medicine kit.

Wilderness Medicine References

The following important references are provided for those who are interested in more thoroughly studying this subject. (The mailing address of the publisher is noted in parentheses after the reference.) There are scores of other references in the medical literature, far too numerous to list in this booklet.

Auerbach, P., and E. Geehr. *Management of Wilderness and Environmental Emergencies*, 2nd edition. Mosby-Year Book, Inc., 1989. (11830 Westline Industrial Drive, P.O. Box 46908, St. Louis, MO 63146.)

Drummond, R. *Ticks*. Berkeley: Wilderness Press, 1990. (2440 Bancroft Way, Berkeley, CA 94704.)

Hackett, P. *Mountain Sickness: Prevention, Recognition, and Treatment*. New York: American Alpine Club, 1989. (113 E. 90th St., New York, NY 10028.)

Houston, C. *Going Higher--The Story of Man and Altitude*. Boston: Little, Brown, and Co., 1987. (34 Beacon St., Boston, MA 02108.)

_____. *High Altitude Physiology Study*. Arlington: Arctic Institute of North America, 1982. (3426 N. Washington Ave, Arlington, VA, 22201.)

Larson, P., and Lane Larson. *Sierra Club Naturalist's Guide to the Deserts of the Southwest*. San Francisco: Sierra Club Books, 1977. (Out of print 1992; excellent section on desert medicine.)

Parcel, G. *Basic Emergency Care of the Sick and Injured*, 4th edition. St. Louis: C. V. Mosby Company, 1990. (11830 Westline Industrial Drive, St. Louis, MO 63141.)

Russell, F. *Snake Venom Poisoning*. Philadelphia: J. B. Lippincott, revised edition 1983. (E. Washington

Square, Philadelphia, PA 19105.)

Wilkerson, J., C. Bangs, and J. Hayward. *Hypothermia, Frostbite, and Other Cold Injuries.* Seattle: The Mountaineers, 1986. (306 2nd Ave. W., Seattle, WA 98119.)

Wilkerson, J. *et al. Medicine for Mountaineering.* 4th edition in press--should be in print later in 1992. Seattle: The Mountaineers. (306 2nd Ave. W., Seattle, WA 98119.)

Emergency Care Products Catalog. Dynamed, 1992. (6300 Yarrow Drive, Carlsbad, CA 92009.)

Emergency Care and Transportation of the Sick and Injured, 5th edition. Chicago: American Academy of Orthopedic Surgeons, 1992. (444 N. Michigan Ave., Chicago, IL 60611.)

Guide for Adult Immunization, 2nd edition. Philadelphia: American College of Physicians, 1990. (4200 Pine St., Philadelphia, PA 19104.)

Journal of Wilderness Medicine. The Wilderness Medical Society. (P. O. Box 2463, Indianapolis, IN 46202.)

The Medical Letter. 56 Harrison St., New Rochelle, New York 10801.

University of Washington *MEDICINE* Vol. 5, No. 2. University of Washington, Seattle, 1978. (Health Sciences Information Services E-307 H. S. C., SC-60, Seattle, WA 98195.)

Wilderness and Rural Life Support Guidelines, Koester, R. J., Editor. dbS Productions. (P.O. Box 1894, Charlottesville, VA 22903.)

Index

About the Author

Fred T. Darvill, Jr., M.D. is a certified specialist in Internal Medicine, a Fellow of the American College of Physicians, a clinical faculty member at the University of Washington School of Medicine, and the author of a number of original research papers on medical subjects. More, he is a dedicated conservationist, an accomplished mountain climber, an experienced wilderness traveller, and the author of a number of books about the North Cascade Mountains in the state of Washington. He has served as medical advisor to, and chairman of, the Skagit Mountain Rescue Unit, is a member of the Medical Committee of the American Alpine Club, and is a contributor to *Medicine for Mountaineering*, edited by Dr. James Wilkerson.

This book is a synthesis of the two loves of Dr. Darvill's life, medicine and the mountains. In the wilderness, special conditions of weather, terrain, time and distance modify routine approaches to illness and accidents. By virtue of his familiarity with both areas, Dr. Darvill is ideally qualified to outline the excellent care recommended in this booklet.

—William R. Halliday, M.D.,
author of *American Caves and Caving*